5 DAYS TO A FLATTER STOMACH

5

days to
a flatter
stomach

MONICA GRENFELL

BⓍXTREE

ACKNOWLEDGEMENTS

I am grateful to the following for their
assistance and advice during the research for this book:

FIONA GEARY MCSP, SRP, DipMDT
Spinal therapy and sports physiotherapist

SHARON McAULEY Dip.I.O.N.
Nutritionist, Inglewood Health Hydro, Berkshire

ADVICE TO THE READER
Before following any medical or dietary advice contained in
this book, it is recommended that you consult your doctor if
you suffer from any health problems or special conditions or
are in any doubt as to its suitability.

First published 1997 by Boxtree, an imprint of Macmillan Publishers Ltd,
25 Eccleston Place, London SW1W 9NF, Basingstoke and Oxford
Associated companies throughout the world
www.macmillan.co.uk

ISBN 0 7522 2130 2

9 10

A CIP catalogue entry for this book is available from the British Library

Typeset by SX Composing DTP, Rayleigh, Essex
Printed by Mackays of Chatham plc, Chatham, Kent
Designed by Hammond Hammond

CONTENTS

Introduction

*H*ow much do you really want a flatter stomach? Maybe you've been fighting the battle for years as you embark on yet another diet and sign on for another punishing round of exercise classes. It all seems to work well for a while, but can you honestly keep it up for good? Although you've always lost weight, is your stomach really any flatter? It can sometimes seem such an uphill struggle that by the end of the day most of us say 'to hell with it', curl up on the sofa and sob into the chocolate box.

If low-fat, high-fibre diets work, why isn't everybody slim? You can diet the Japanese way, the Florida way, detoxify your body or combine your food. You can sit with a calculator working out fat units and calorie totals, but at the end of the day can you really say you've won? And why do most slimming club champions regain all the weight they've lost?

'I always go back to my old eating habits', one lapsed slimmer lamented, and that says it all. It's not food that makes you fat, it's the way you eat it, and the amount. If you've been striving for years to get a flatter stomach and given up hope, hang on. It doesn't come easily and you need determination, but it's not as hard as you think. I've helped thousands of women to get slim, and my methods always work.

During the past decade we've been told we can 'have it all', but there has been a high price to pay. Yes, women could dominate the boardroom and have a body to die for. We could hone ourselves to perfection and feel proud of our defined shoulder muscles, but at the end of the day we've been too exhausted from all that step aerobics and too washed out and irritable from not eating to enjoy the benefits of looking good. The stress just isn't worth it, and if you're the type of woman who can only enjoy a chocolate eclair if you can go and work it off at aerobics, this diet isn't for you. Let's face it, there must be an easier way to have your cake and eat it.

In the romance stakes, men don't fall for our fat ratios. A good figure and bags of confidence are what get us noticed, combined with a relaxed, easy attitude to food. It's no good inspiring awe in your friends if you're terrified of a slice of cheese.

In the new age of femininity, hours spent burning calories are out. Treating yourself like a second-class citizen with fat-free alternatives while the rest of the family eats the real thing is also passé. As we come up to the new millennium we can wave goodbye to oppressive regimes and hard, manly torsos, and welcome back a few curves. But the new relaxed attitude doesn't mean we can afford to let ourselves go. Daily exercise has always been your best beauty aid and a flawless skin and shiny hair depend on good eating habits. For the first time I have taken the stress out of slimming and put back reality. Reality means food people really want to eat. Reality means not having to spend ten minutes packing a holdall full of equipment and changing into special gear just to go and exercise. Reality means admitting that we just don't want to eat all that bran.

The way we feel about our weight and size can dominate our lives. We can be irritable all day simply because we woke up feeling fat. Just like a Bad Hair Day, a Fat Stomach Day is awful, especially if you particularly wanted to look your best. 'She's as slim as anything', one man said to me recently about his wife, 'and I think she's gorgeous, but if I try to put my arms round her she pulls away and says she's fat. I definitely can't go anywhere near her stomach! Are all women like that?' I'm afraid we are.

I have been advising women about their figures for many years, and one thing is obvious – most women are not hugely fat. Many would simply like to lose the odd stone or a few pounds, but when they reach their target weight they're still unhappy about their shape, which is the real frustration after putting such a lot of effort into the diet. Although too much fat coupled with poor muscle tone are undoubtedly the main causes of a large stomach, very often the problem is also the *type* of food eaten, the *time and frequency* of eating and the *way* the food is eaten.

BUT I NEED TO LOSE A COUPLE OF STONE!
Don't worry. The 5-day plan is intended to get you started and

to introduce you to a new way of eating. Thereafter The Maintenance Plan will keep you losing weight steadily and safely. The point about this flatter stomach plan is that you eat little and often, with NO low-fat, low-calorie or sugar-free alternatives, and once you have lost a little weight and can fit into smaller clothes you'll have your confidence. Five days is enough to show you real results which you'll be delighted with.

Believe me, if you've been on diets before, this diet is *completely different!*

Are you serious?

'A flatter stomach in only 5 days! Are you serious?' That was the response of several people when I told them I was writing this book, but then I introduced them to my old client Sally, who'd done the whole plan a year after her hysterectomy. Having always been lovely and slim, at the age of only thirty-nine she'd started to put weight on alarmingly quickly after her operation, and despite hormonal treatment she knew the real reason was her constant yo-yo dieting pattern. 'This lady did it', I told them. 'Meet Sally, who was in a desperate state about her stomach when we met. Sally, tell them how it worked for you.'

Sally beamed. 'It worked – honestly' she said, patting her slim size 10 figure. 'I was so depressed about my weight and I'd have done anything. None of my clothes fitted. I started rigid dieting and would go all day on just fruit, then have a big main meal. By the end of a few days I felt slimmer, but I was so hungry I'd start on the fridge.' Sally laughed at the memory. 'I didn't exactly binge, but I'd eat masses. Then I'd just reckon that I'd done so much damage I might as well eat as much as I could. Of course the next day a new diet would start, I'd go off and swim twenty lengths and the whole thing began again.'

Sally was sceptical about the diet when she first saw the meal plans, and was sure she'd gain weight.

'I wasn't used to eating so many times a day, and I almost said no. Then I thought "well, it's only five days", so I agreed.' She smiled. 'I'm so glad I did. I lost 5lb, which I know is mainly water, but I was retaining a lot of fluid which made me feel bloated, so when I got rid of that and felt slimmer I wasn't tempted to binge.' She went on to lose 12lb over four weeks on The Maintenance Plan, she toned up and now pays a lot of attention to her posture.

Sally's story is typical. I had been putting clients through the diet for years, and was confident about its success rate, but then I decided to do a fair and balanced test. After all, people might just want to please me, so how about finding a group of total strangers?

I appealed for volunteers on local radio stations around the country, in the *Swindon Evening Advertiser* newspaper in which I write a weekly health and fitness column, and I advertised in women's magazines. I also contacted friends and family who worked in large organizations up and down the country, and they soon came up with lists of women who were keen to give it a go. I was inundated with volunteers, but in the end I selected just 200 people to go on the plan.

Nobody had any idea of what the plan was aiming to achieve only that I was testing a diet and exercise plan for a book. They all kept diaries for me, as I was interested not only in weight loss and figure improvement, but also if the meals worked, whether their families enjoyed them and whether they could find the foods easily. It is no good suggesting a regime which puts people to endless trouble, or food which nobody can take to the workplace.

The detailed responses of some of the team are contained in the next section although I could not include all of them, much as I would have liked to. However, the collected diaries showed:

All the testers lost weight, even the most sceptical

All the testers felt noticeably and pleasingly slimmer

All the testers had managed to give up any laxatives and stomach medicines they had been taking for wind, and were thrilled at how calming the diet was

All the testers said they could happily stick with the regime

All the testers said they were pleased and relieved to be able to eat 'proper' food again – such as butter, eggs and cheese.

Nobody disliked the diet in any way

I believe I cannot go better than the evidence of those 200 volunteers who were so kind as to put themselves through my 5-day regime and my grateful thanks go out to them all. Don't be sceptical. If you can have such a result in only five days, think what you can achieve in a month!

5 MEALS A DAY!
HOW MANY CALORIES WILL I BE EATING?

Your 5 meals each day will consist of two more substantial meals and three light meals. The calorie counts of the larger meals are anywhere between 200–400 calories, and the light meals range from 100–200 calories. There are two or three choices for your meals, to take into account your preferences for plain or fancier food, and all the recipes with their calorie contents are to be found at the back of the book.

The reasons people don't stick with a diet

Here are some of the reasons people give up a diet, and my solutions:

1. You don't see results quickly enough

Crash diets used to be a quick way of losing weight and cheering yourself up, but they didn't work in the long term because it wasn't fat which was lost, but water, and there was little appreciable difference to your figure. After a week or so you went back to your old eating habits and all the weight piled back on again. Well, that won't happen on this plan. Seeing and feeling a difference quickly is a major psychological boost, which is why the 5-day plan works so well. It is The Maintenance Plan that ensures you will stick with the diet in the weeks ahead. If you're already planning your summer holiday, now's the time to start.

This isn't a crash diet, but the first results are swift. You will also significantly reduce bloating and improve your muscle tone, both of which will increase your confidence.

2. You reach a plateau, and there doesn't seem to be any point

This happens to everybody. I can promise you that if you stay with it and carry on with the diet, the weight will suddenly fall off again. DON'T give in and eat all the wrong things again. Your body is simply adjusting to your new metabolism. Don't panic.

3. You have to make one meal for yourself and another for the rest of the family

My meal suggestions can be enjoyed by everyone. I don't use ANY low-calorie or low-fat alternatives, but some recipes are adapted to reduce thoughtless and liberal use of fattening ingredients. There's no need to treat yourself as a second-class citizen just because you're on a diet. We all appreciate quality, and that means decent butter, cheese and real cream. As a guide, ask yourself what kind of dessert you'd give to a guest? The lowest-calorie variety or the richest? Many of the meals on this diet are standard favourites, which old and young alike can enjoy.

4. You feel hungry all the time

On this diet you'll eat five or six times a day. The secret of slimness is to eat *regularly* in *small amounts*. Ever woken at 3am feeling bright and wide awake, only to fall asleep and wake at 7am feeling dead? This is classic low blood sugar. Taking a late evening snack gives you a restful sleep from which you wake refreshed.

5. You feel washed out and tired

You won't feel tired because the frequent meals keep your blood sugar level up and provide plenty of starch.

6. You have to weigh everything and count calories

You need to weigh some things, but generally we do it by spoonfuls and portion control. Once you get the hang of it you'll soon know how much something weighs, and it doesn't do to get hung up about every gram.

7. You feel bloated on all that fruit and fibre

Fruit and fibre are undoubtedly important, but they can cause terrible bloating, which is no good when you want to feel your best. Feeling bloated doesn't do anything for your confidence, so high-bran breakfasts are OUT. We will be eating soluble fibre and plenty of starchy foods during the day, and keeping high-fibre snacks until the evening when they can do less damage.

All diets work for a while. After that, we fall back into our old eating habits. People who seem to eat anything that they want and stay slim eat regularly, they eat when they are hungry and they stop when they are full. It isn't as simple as saying that people with weight problems eat too much. They eat for the wrong reasons, they eat beyond the point at which they have had enough and they eat erratically. Eating the right or wrong foods isn't really the issue here, because the key is the amount we eat and the discipline of mealtimes.

DISCIPLINE IS LIBERATING

In its own way, disciplining yourself is liberating. All the stress of deciding what and when to eat, the huge ranges of choices, the ability to eat now or in two hours; time – this is why people have weight problems. By deciding for you, I have taken on all the responsibility, thereby leaving you free to relax and to get on with other things.

IT WORKED FOR ME

I devised the diet because it worked for me. As a fitness professional, I have spent years standing in front of exercise classes wearing a figure-hugging leotard and leggings, with a roomful of women studying every bulge and wobbly bit. I used to half starve to stay slim, then I started to eat five times a day and didn't gain an ounce! The secret was plenty of starch and smaller meals, and the best thing has been the flat stomach. I believe in this way of eating and exercising. I have put many clients through the plan and I know it will work for you.

YOU'LL BE SO MUCH MORE CONFIDENT

A good figure and a flat stomach are worth having because they give us confidence. You don't want to be covering yourself up and choosing clothes you don't really want to wear. You've already made the decision to do something about your stomach by buying this book, but I also want you to continue the plan into the future. If going on a diet and exercising are difficult for you, remember that you're going to get your rewards. I have made the exercise routine easy for you to follow without having to go out to the gym every day. I have devised a meal plan which is quick and uncomplicated. There's no reason for you not to achieve your flatter stomach before the week's out!

BEING REALISTIC ABOUT YOUR LIFESTYLE

If you go out to work and have a family to organize, it is unlikely that you will want to come home to cook a fancy recipe requiring a long list of ingredients, half of which end up rotting at the back of the fridge. If you're vainly struggling through winter trying to block up draughts and peel potatoes with your coat on, you won't thank me if I suggest a cottage cheese salad and frozen sorbet for supper. Well, on this diet there's something to suit everyone, from hearty porridge to spicy chilli to sophisticated smoked salmon pasta.

5 BASIC FOODS

With just 5 basic foods, plus additions to make them into nourishing and balanced meals, you won't have to worry about endless choices.

5 DAYS AND 5 EXERCISES

It's vital that you exercise those stomach muscles every day. Set aside three to five periods in the day when you can exercise for just five minutes as a bare minimum – if you can manage more that's great. The danger is setting yourself too high a goal. If you start on day one promising yourself an hour a day of aerobics, you'll only feel a failure if you can't manage it. I have kept the stomach exercises to five variations, all of which tone and trim your abdominal muscles effectively while you are dieting.

5 POSTURE STRETCHES

However good your muscles are, however slim you've become, if you stand and sit badly your stomach will hang out. Every day has five easy stretches to maintain a good body alignment, which will make you appear inches slimmer.

NO SUBSTITUTES

'I can't believe I'll be eating butter!' said one of my testers. 'My last diet banned cheese completely' said another, adding that a lifetime without her favourite cheese and pickle sandwich wouldn't be worth living. I agree. But what about the fat content of this diet?

In the past ten years the nation has been low-fat mad, so how do we account for the fact that obesity is at an all-time high, I wonder? And why are so many low-fat addicts still fat?

The fact is, people will never stop eating fatty diets, and nobody sticks with a menu plan stuffed with healthy alternatives. The alternatives are not healthy, indeed they're usually crammed with so many additives the list takes up half the packaging. Yes, my diet insists on proper butter, *crème fraîche*, cheese and eggs, but when most of the population has been existing on a diet of crisps, hot dogs, kilos of toffees, ice-cream and pizzas, washed down with lager or fizzy drinks, this diet is the healthiest some people will have been eating for years!

TWO-SPEED DIET CHOICE

Your diet plan comes in two speeds:
i) The Standard 5-day Diet
ii) The Maintenance Diet

The Standard Plan is very specific about what to eat and when, it bans alcohol, chocolate, cakes and biscuits, and it guarantees fantastic results. The Maintenance Diet, on the other hand, offers slightly more choice from the recipe section, a few sweet snacks and alcohol. If you want to know how to keep up the good eating habits you've learned, this diet offers more meal choices and variety, and you'll continue to lose weight steadily.

In addition, there's a section on vegetarian meals, although most of the recipes can be easily adapted.

5 DAYS TO A FLATTER STOMACH

Half the battle is your determination. Going for a few walks and eating smaller meals isn't hard, but if you're in love with the great indoors and your local takeaway, it's going to take a shift in attitude until you train yourself to think differently. But DO keep at it. Nobody was ever sorry she lost weight. Nobody ever looked back wistfully to her fat days. *Good luck!*

Success stories

My whole weight-loss concept is so different from most diets, I wanted to put a team of testers through it. Not just to see if it worked, because I knew that it would, but to see if it was practical. After all, it's no good going through a punishing regime if the rest of the family suffer, and nobody wants a sandwich lunch which is soggy by the time you get to work. I put the word out around the country for women as far apart as Kent, Nottingham and Perth to join in the diet and exercise plan, and they all reported fantastic results.

I chose a cross-section of people. A couple of women wanted to lose at least two stone apiece, several testers reported few problems with their weight, but despair with their stomachs after having babies, and the majority simply wanted to lose about 7–10lb and tone up their muscles. They all kept diaries for me, and I'm delighted to report that their results exceeded even my own wildest expectations. Here is a selection of their verdicts:

Irene Norton, forty-two, a medical secretary in Faversham, Kent, is married with four teenage children
'I had to let you know straight away how completely thrilled I was with the diet. I needed to lose more than a stone, but I find conventional diets too long-winded and not really practical for long-term use.

At first I thought "Five days! I'll believe it when I see it!", but because my problem has always been psychological – I suppose I want instant success or I get disheartened – this was the perfect plan for me because I *felt* so much slimmer by the end of just three days, and that spurred me on.

I had to give up the diet for a long weekend because we went away for a wedding, and I realized how awful I'd always felt before. It's the bloating I think, and when your stomach's wrong you feel wrong all over. I've now gone back to the diet and have kept to it for four weeks now, lost 12lb and gone down a dress size and many inches.

To tell the truth I couldn't care less about what the scales say, I'm more interested in how my clothes look, and my eldest daughter said yesterday that I looked ten years younger now I'm back to cinching in my waist with a nice belt.

I'm really proud of my figure now, the diet's wonderful and I'll keep on the maintenance plan for good. It's nice to have someone spell it all out for you.'

Maria Telling, eighteen, is single and a sociology student at Manchester University

'The exercises worked best for me. I'm very untoned as I'm lazy about exercise, and my stomach had got quite flabby. Knowing there was only five minutes of exercising meant that I wasn't reluctant to do it, although I did tell myself I simply MUST do it three times a day. It wasn't easy, but the thing was, it worked! I didn't believe that you could do so much without going to an aerobics class for an hour a time, but I can honestly say that after five days I had an entirely different shape. I hold myself better too and I think that's made a huge difference.

As far as the food was concerned, it was perfect. I'm sharing a flat which has an ancient oven and only two electric rings, so anything complicated was obviously out. I've also got no money! I spent far less on this diet than I usually do eating at the subsidized refectory at college, and my favourite meal was the chilli con carne because we could all share it, and it cost about £4 for four of us, which was brilliant.'

Siobhan Everitt, thirty, is married with three children under five

'I wanted to lose about half a stone and have tried a lot of diets, but this is the first one I'd stuck with. I suffer from Irritable Bowel Syndrome, which blows me out, but with this diet I was so much better with less wind and grumbling feelings. I think it was because it wasn't just fruit, fruit, fruit, which always makes me feel quite empty.

I have to work hard at keeping slim because with three children there's always the wrong food around and you're always making something. I tend to eat all the wrong things too. I'll have a Mars bar in the afternoon because I'm starving, then I'll think "oh, I can't have any tea because I ate that chocolate", so then I'm hungry again in the evening and eat a load of biscuits, so really it's a lot of rubbish I'm eating. And so it goes on.

With this diet the food is so enjoyable. For the first time I'm eating quite a lot, and with five meals a day I feel I'm not deprived. Most diets don't allow eating between meals, so they're hard to stick to over a long period. You tell us we can eat a snack if we feel like it, so I don't feel guilty.

The meals were really easy to prepare. With three young children I haven't time to mess about. On other diets you have to buy new things and you're making up all this waffle, just for something on your plate. I'd prefer to stick with shepherd's pie!

I loved the avocado pear. I've never eaten one before and I thought "oh, I'm not sure about this, but it's on the diet", so I tried it, with the prawns. It was wonderful!

I'm carrying on with the diet from now on. I lost 4lb and my stomach seems so much slimmer. I won't eat the old way ever again.'

Gillian Jaworsky, thirty-five, is an actress, married, no children and living in Wandsworth

'I admit to being obsessed with my body, and I notice every millimetre on it. My husband and I entertain, so I was a bit worried I'd be either stuck with ghastly hotpots or have to give up the diet altogether when we entertained. How wrong I was! I could eat smoked salmon and *crème fraîche* and the cheese soufflé was out of this world!

I'm an intermittent, picky eater. I also binge then starve for days because I feel wretched. I suppose it's because I'm in the theatre and my job means looking good and it's quite stressful. I tend to go for three days being good, then I eat a square of chocolate and think I might as well eat the bar. Then I hate myself so much I have two or three slices of cake which I don't even fancy. Anyway, I was thrilled to be asked to test a new diet, and even more thrilled to say that I ate quite normally – which for me seemed a lot – and I even lost two pounds in the five days. I think it's marvellous.'

Gillian Frame, forty three, dental receptionist from Keighley, North Yorkshire, is a divorced mother of four children
'I am very particular about how I look, especially as I've joined a dating agency recently and am going out regularly to meet new men. I needed to tone up a bit and probably should lose about a stone.

On my other diets, if I went out I was terrified of having a pat of butter with my bread and I'd ask for any sauce to be left off. On this diet I felt completely liberated! It's difficult to describe, but I now just say yes to everything. As I've learnt to eat dainty amounts and not to worry that I'll never eat a square meal again, I feel as if all the tension of a diet has gone. I've done the diet now for three weeks and have lost half a stone, and the best thing is that I feel I'm not on a diet at all.

I invited one man I met over to my house and cooked him the spaghetti with smoked salmon and dill. It took me about ten minutes start to finish, and he was going mad, saying how fantastic it was and that I must have been slaving away for hours. I didn't say anything!

I just can't believe how toned I feel, and how flat my stomach is. I was really, really unsure of it when I was asked, but now I'm telling all my friends. My children all eat exactly the same as me, too, and as one of my daughters has quite a weight problem I'm pleased that she's losing weight too.'

Helen Foster, thirty-one, a unit trust dealer, lives with her partner
'My porridge breakfast filled me up so much I almost didn't need my mid-morning snack every day, but I ate it and wasn't so hungry by lunchtime.

I haven't much of a weight problem, but I'm always holding my stomach in. I didn't think I'd get used to the amount of food – usually I tend to pig-out when I get home from work as I'm so hungry, but eating a mid-afternoon snack put paid to that. I could happily go right through until dinner and eat far less.

I managed to fit in several sessions of stomach exercises, although it wasn't easy at the office. I decided to do five minutes of exercises in the morning and again on my return from work, and I did three aerobics classes too!

By day five I was definitely into the swing of it. At first I thought I would be hungry, especially at night, but it seems that I'm eating most of the time and I lost 3lb by day four. I'm sure I've lost about 1in off my hips! On day five I put on a skirt which I always use for testing my size and it felt quite roomy! Great!

I'm starting The Maintenance Diet next week because I'm off on my holiday and I'll want to have a few drinks and sweet things but not undo all the good work I've just done. Then when I come back I'll start The Standard Diet again, in case I've gained any weight. I know I haven't got a real figure problem, but my stomach drives me mad and I'm always hiding it. This diet has been just wonderful, I think I'll stay on it for good.

Marian Crawford, thirty-seven, is a housewife with three children

'I'm tall, 5ft 10in, and I was stick-thin before I had the children. It's my stomach that gets me down, I feel I can take in tucks at the sides! Having children has been like blowing up a balloon, keeping it there all Christmas and letting it down again – it never goes back to what it was before, does it?

I needed to tone up, and I found the best help were the stomach exercises. I've also got terrible insides. I'm on the go all day with the children and two new little puppies, and I don't often eat much from breakfast to teatime. I was taking vitamins because I was tired, then laxatives because I was constipated! On this diet I managed to give all that up. My stomach was less grumbly and felt much flatter, and I'm pleased I haven't got all that bloatedness now.

I never used to drink much water or eat much fruit, and now I will as it's sorted my problems out. I looked at the diet sheet and thought "there's so much food – I'll put on weight", but I lost 4lb and wasn't hungry for a minute. I'll definitely keep it up.'

Janet and Simon Ashworth, fifty-one and fifty, are both nurses at a Nottingham hospital and have grown-up children
(Janet) 'We decided to go on the diet together, for support. Simon wouldn't have gone on any of my other diets (which I'm always starting!) because he says the food's too finicky, but when he saw omelettes, mashed potatoes and roast chicken his eyes lit up.

I must admit I was a bit sceptical about adding *crème fraîche* to one dish and cooking something else in butter, but after all the years I've been on these low-fat spreads, good old butter was fantastic. I know you can't have lashings of it, but somehow knowing that you're eating the real thing makes you go easy on it anyway. It was like pure gold!

I suppose I'm quite overweight – about two and a half stone – and Simon's the same. I've been dieting for as long as I can remember, but what puts me off is calculating the portions, measuring each out and then piling on the vegetables because you can't eat again for hours. This diet was such common sense because you just eat small amounts of everything.

My dress is much looser round my stomach, and I reckon to have lost two inches, although I can't have, can I? I'm staying on the regular diet for another two weeks, then I'll go on to The Maintenance Diet.'

(Simon) 'I joined Janet to support her, thinking I'd hate it. In fact I've lost weight too. I feel much, much smaller in my abdomen, and far brighter and healthier. I don't know what it is, but I'm really bouncing around now. I've managed to give up my morning chocolate bar with no cravings, and no diet's ever got me to do that!

My favourite meal was the chilli con carne which I hadn't eaten before – well I had, but it had tasted quite fatty. This seemed rather plain while I was making it, but it tasted lovely.

It was hard at first, I'll admit, to look at a small saucer of salad or a couple of spoons of veggies, but you soon want much less. I tried to eat a piece of fish and three potatoes today and had to stop after two of them, I was so full. I think this diet's the best thing that's ever happened to us.'

Louise Cordas, twenty-seven, is married with one child and another on the way

'I actually lost four stone to get married! Then I put it back on, got pregnant and thought there wasn't any point. After Matthew was born I knew I should diet, but in the back of my mind was the thought that I knew we wanted two children quite close together and there wouldn't be any point in dieting only to get pregnant again.

I started the diet just before I fell pregnant with this one, so obviously I've given it up for a bit, but I'll start it straight away after the birth. I totally believe in this diet. The main thing I like is that I can give my little boy anything I have to eat, which isn't the case with some fancy diet books with all their exotic menus. I never felt hungry, but I knew that if I did I could eat a banana or a slice of toast and not even think about it. I loved the pasta primavera. The pesto sauce and the *crème fraîche* were completely yummy, and it only took a few minutes. All the ingredients were in the local supermarket, so I got everything there and didn't have to traipse around for bits.

I can't wait to go back on it and lose all this weight again.'

Dee Whittaker, forty-eight, a beauty therapist, is widowed with two adult daughters

'Although I'm a beauty therapist I've let myself go since my husband died. I always used to play badminton and swim, but the exercise went out of the window last year when I felt so depressed. My weight soared and I couldn't do anything about it.

I've lost 4lb and feel about a stone lighter after a week on this diet – I extended it to a week because I didn't want to stop. I actually found the posture section most revealing – I didn't realize until I caught sight of myself in a shop window that I was slouching so badly. My neck was all scrunched up and my chest seemed to sink into my stomach! I think about it all the time now, and it's made my stomach hold itself in and look controlled, which has made me look more confident, my friend tells me.

I thought that exercising several times a day would be a chore, but I started to look forward to it. It was like sending myself on a course. I felt I had homework to do several times a day. Each page of the diet was like Monica talking to me and encouraging me, and the best encouragement was that she said it had worked for her.

I don't want to stop. I feel I can adapt the ideas for myself now, which is the idea of The Maintenance Plan. It starts off seeming weird with all that mashed potato, rice pudding and bananas, and I didn't think I'd like bio-yoghurt until I put stewed fruit into it. I'd recommend this diet plan to anyone of any age. My stomach's much, much flatter, and I've got my confidence back.'

Sally Pallister, twenty-three, a journalist for a woman's magazine, is single and lives in Sheffield

'My life is one mad rush from the beginning of the day to the end, and I go for long hours without eating. Then when I do, it's all the wrong things. I grab a sandwich or stop at one of the local bistros for a snack which is usually a burger or curry, then I feel completely blown up for hours. I also sit at my word processor for sometimes six hours without a break, and my bottom was spreading. I weighed about 10lb too much and my figure was a disgrace for someone my age, but I thought, "what can I do?"

If I hadn't been asked to be a tester I wouldn't have bothered with a diet, but when I saw the meals all written out for me it took away the responsibility and I said yes straight away. I'm so glad I did.

What I liked was the simplicity. I suppose you'd call me a typical career girl because I'm always out, and my new cooker which I've had for six months is still in its cellophane! I haven't got a freezer either, so it would have been no good if I'd needed frozen stuff. The food was the type anyone would like, with no preparation if you didn't want to and it really worked. After the five days I was 4lb lighter, but I felt really quite svelte. My stomach had lost all its hugeness and I didn't need to hold it in all the time. I did do the exercises too, which was an effort for me as I hate exercise, but as it was only a few minutes here and there I thought it was worth it. Frankly, I didn't think so few exercises would make a difference, but they have.

I've decided to stick with the 5-day plan every Monday to Friday and as I have a hectic social life at weekends I'll do my own thing then, though I won't go overboard. I'd recommend the diet to any of my friends. It doesn't assume you're half of a couple or have 2.4 kids, as all recipes are for one person.'

Molly Agnew, seventy-eight, is a retired headmistress living in Cheshire

'I've always been careful about my appearance, and just because I'm retired it doesn't mean I've given up. I still like to wear tailored clothes and I have a lot of Christmas engagements this year.

The diet worked a treat. My stomach's more delicate than it used to be and I can't take too many spices or fibre. The starch was somehow calming and I've just worn a skirt I haven't fitted into for 10 years!'

Linda Thompson, forty, an assistant recruitment manager in the NHS, is married with two children

'I'm a lifetime member of the diet club, and at the moment I'd say my weight's stable. I lost 3lb on the diet, and my friend who did it with me lost a good inch off her stomach in only five days!

I really liked the fact that when I started work at 9am I knew I didn't have to wait long before I could have a snack. I couldn't have gone on until lunchtime.

We eat late in the evening at home, so I saved the main meal until 9pm. I particularly liked the fish content of the diet and I would definitely stick with The Maintenance Plan. I think it was a great diet, and it was nice to see results so quickly. I never knew there were so many additives in the diet foods I'd been eating – it really makes you think, doesn't it?'

1

5 days

5 common problems

Y ou have five days and just one goal in mind – a flatter stomach. We are going to tackle this together by looking at what causes our stomachs to be big in the first place.

1. **You are carrying too much fat**
2. **Your stomach is constantly bloated**
3. **You suffer from constipation**
4. **Your muscles need toning**
5. **Your posture is terrible**

Now let's look at each of these causes, and see what can be done about them:

> **1. YOU ARE CARRYING TOO MUCH FAT ON YOUR STOMACH**

All women carry some fat on their stomachs and hips. 'Mother Nature' doesn't know that you've decided not to have children or have finished raising your family. If you are a normal female in her reproductive years, the only aim of Nature is to ensure that even if you are starving, you still have enough fat supplies to maintain a pregnancy. Those supplies are typically anywhere between 17 per cent and 26 per cent of your body mass. If your fat supplies fall dangerously low, which can happen through illness or severe dieting, Nature will see to it that you cannot conceive – by stopping your periods. An example is the elite gymnast who has to have very little body fat, or the anorexic, both of whom find that their periods have stopped until they gain weight. Because of this need to support life, the last fat stores to go are those which protect our reproductive areas and that means our lower body area. Unfortunately this leads to the perennial problem which most of us complain about, namely fat on the hips and abdomen, which seems to remain, stubbornly, despite our most heroic efforts to shift it. However, what we must aim to do is to reduce excess fat deposits which have come about by eating too much food and taking too little exercise.

BEATING THE CRAVINGS

If we're not allowed something, we crave it all the more. Look at people who appear to eat anything they like, and see what they actually eat. Because they allow themselves anything they fancy it loses its forbidden appeal. Slim people stop when they've had enough to eat. Having tasted a delicacy, they don't feel they have to have more and more of it, and they rarely have the attitude of 'I've paid for it, I might as well eat it'. Any food left over will go into the bin. If you eat food to save wasting it, it has gone in your internal bin.

YOU CAN ALWAYS GO BACK FOR MORE

Wasting food is wrong, but why put too much on your plate in the first place? You can always go back for more. Try this trick for controlling your food intake and see if it works. Put out your evening meal (or lunch, if this is your main cooked meal) and immediately *halve* it. Cut everything exactly in two, and place the second portion on a clean plate to refrigerate. Tell yourself you're going to eat one plate now and the other plate in one hour's time. I have tried this with countless people and most of them find they don't want the second plateful, or if they do, it saves them from another snack. Try it.

'UNLIMITED' FOODS

Most diets give you an 'unlimited' foods list. This is to say that if you have not had enough to eat, you can pile your plate as high as you like with something else. It also means that when you are restricted to three meals a day and no snacks, you'll take every opportunity to eat masses of anything you're allowed during one of those precious meals. The concept of 'unlimited' foods encourages gluttony. If you have a problem with food, you must learn to eat smaller, daintier meals. On my diet, nothing is unlimited.

SOME OF THE MOST COMMON REASONS WHY PEOPLE BECOME FAT

a. Eating when bored

Winter is worse than summer for this. Long dark nights mean hours have to be filled and the temptation to flop in front of the television, stoke up the fire and fill a few bowls with crisps is much greater. Better still, why not send for a pizza and garlic bread? Oh, and you could have that lager, why not? After all, there's nothing else to do.

Summer too, has its hazards. If it gets hot you lounge in the garden, unable to summon the energy to pull a few weeds or take the dog for a walk. Lying there panting, it's easy to reach for another fizzy drink or the choc ices. After all, you've just had a day in a steaming office and you deserve a break. Holiday time becomes one long meal, and if it rains on holiday, there's another reason to pile into the nearest teashop for a gigantic cream tea. If you've a problem with food, boredom is your enemy.

b. Eating the wrong things

There's no such thing as a bad food. Not even chocolate or chips or sugar or butter. There are only bad diets. If you confined yourself to steamed fish and spinach to the exclusion of everything else, you would soon be suffering from malnutrition. Indeed, if you were to eat such a diet, the inclusion of the odd pizza and fries would redress the balance nicely, and be exactly what your body would need.

c. Not using up your food intake

Fat settles because your food is surplus to requirements. There's no set amount of food which we can all eat and stay slim. It all depends on our lifestyles and how much energy we use each day, but if you want to eat well and stay slim, you *must* increase your exercise.

d. Metabolic rates and eating too little

It's easy to raise your metabolic rate if you put your mind to it. If you lay in bed doing absolutely nothing for a week, you'd still need about 1,450 calories (1,900 for a man) just to keep your body working, your heart beating, your lungs filling with air and so forth. This is called your **Basal Metabolic Rate (BMR)**. The minute you add any activity at all to this, you increase your calorie needs. You should not decrease your daily calorie intake lower than your BMR.

Eating too little actually makes you gain weight in the long run. Your body is programmed to preserve life, so when your food intake is reduced your metabolism slows down as well. This is not to say that it happens overnight. We all have the odd day of eating very little, in the same way that we sometimes have an indulgent weekend or holiday, but consistent dieting means that when you do eat, the food is stored as fat for an emergency. If you remember that Nature's job is to preserve life at all costs, you are well on the way to understanding why cutting out food in order to stay slim just doesn't work. If you consistently eat irregularly, your metabolism will slow down to preserve your fat supplies, keep you alive as long as possible and allow you to reproduce if necessary. Eating little and often serves the dual purpose of preventing weight gain and keeping your metabolism ticking away happily at a moderate rate, so that the calories you have taken in are burnt efficiently.

---

2. YOUR STOMACH IS CONSTANTLY BLOATED

Is this your problem? Talking to a friend the other day who is slim and quite tall, she complained '...my stomach's nice and flat first thing in the morning but by six o'clock I've a job to hold it in. It's embarrassing. I know I need to lose weight, but I feel too self-conscious to wear a leotard at Keep Fit.'

Does this sound like you? Almost everyone I meet in my slimming clinic seems to have suffered from this problem at some time or another, and it can cause much misery being overweight. Indeed, many slightly overweight women who *don't* have a bloating problem and feel that their stomach is nice and flat, often don't worry about their weight at all.

CONTROLLING AND BANISHING THE BLOAT

A large part of this diet concerns avoiding foods which cause irritable bowels and abdominal discomfort. These are the ones you should watch for:

BRAN Unfortunately, in the past twenty years we have become besotted with high-fibre diets. Fibre is undoubtedly necessary, and in the past we have had too little of it to the detriment of our health, but most people think of fibre as being bowls of bran. Bran has no nutritional value, it passes through the system whole and is not digested, causing a 'scrubbing' action in the bowel. The bacteria it produces in the large bowel ferment and produce gas. *Too much bran and other insoluble fibre causes an irritable and gassy stomach*, so it will be restricted.

STRAWBERRIES Strawberries contain a dietary fibre called lignin, which is in the seeds, and which is extremely laxative. We will be eating strawberries for their vitamin C content and their versatility, but they will be restricted to the evening.

CRUCIFEROUS VEGETABLES Cruciferous vegetables are notorious for producing gas and they are restricted on this diet. They include cabbage, Brussels sprouts, cauliflower, broccoli and kale.

PULSES These include peas, all kinds of beans, lentils and sweetcorn. Pulses contain protein, they are low in fat and the starches in them provide a steady source of glucose. They are also cheap to buy and can be used as the basis for a huge range of meals. Pulses are high in fibre because the outer skin or shell cannot be broken down by the body, and it passes through the system whole. On this diet our pulse vegetables will be sweetcorn and peas.

FIZZY DRINKS Fizzy drinks are not included in this diet. We will be drinking plenty of water, either plain tap or mineral water.

A staggering 12 million people in this country – one in every five – suffers from Irritable Bowel Syndrome (IBS), a condition which causes untold stress and unhappiness to sufferers. IBS is not the only cause of bloating, discomfort and painful wind, but the term covers a multitude of problems, most of which are little understood by the medical profession.

People who go to the doctor because they have abdominal cramps, alternating diarrhoea and constipation and flatulence, which appear to be out of proportion with the rest of their general health, usually fear some terrible disease or cancer. They go through a battery of tests, all of which prove negative, and the doctor is forced to the conclusion that the symptoms are unexplained. A chat on stress and food intolerance is the next step, with a possible referral to a dietician. High fibre is usually recommended, although in many cases this only makes the problem worse. Another cause of food intolerance is eating TOO MUCH of the same food – for example having fifteen apples a day or eight bananas – which can make your stomach start to react against it.

SO WHAT DO YOU DO IF BLOATING IS CAUSED BY FOOD INTOLERANCE?

There is no big mystery about food intolerance. We are all human, and some things don't agree with us as well as others. The simple solution is to leave them out. Remember that the normal digestive process causes all sorts of grumblings and rumblings which are nothing to be alarmed about, and do not necessarily mean that the food you have eaten is doing you any harm. I am asking you to avoid certain foods because they can cause bloating, but it *doesn't* mean to say that they are harmful.

If you have no pain or cramping and feel healthy, then try my anti-bloat diet. You might not be aware of how irritating some foods are, however healthy they may be. If you are feeling miserable because you are sloshing around in gallons of fruit juice because you've been told to eat six pieces of fruit a day, or shovelling in food that you don't really like, then don't do it.

If you still have digestive problems after the 5-day plan, or if your problems become more severe while you are following it, see your doctor immediately.

The following foods rarely cause allergic or intolerance reactions (such as bloating and discomfort):

lamb, pears, artichokes, lettuce, carrots, peaches, apples, rice

In my opinion, too many diets recommend vast quantities of fruit and fibre. While unquestionably healthy and nutritious, they nevertheless leave you with an uncomfortable abdomen. No slimming plan can be counted as successful if it leaves you feeling less than confident. Virtue may have its own reward, but if you have managed without your favourite chocolate-chip biscuits and fried eggs for a week, a tight waistband and an inability to hold in your stomach are a pretty poor return.

IBS is a circular problem. Stress is also known to cause bloating. If you are stressed your food isn't digested properly causing cramps and pain. Starting the day by worrying about this possibility only makes it worse.

Most bloating problems are easily sorted out through attention to some small details, and I suggest you spend a day or so trying them out to see if you feel any better.

a. Are you eating too quickly?

'I'm always on the go', said a friend. 'It's all rush in our house first thing, and I shovel a plate of cereal down me in about three minutes. Then at lunch the kids are arguing and I'm trying to prepare the evening meal as well. I just wolf it down, and always feel full later, even if I've only had a sandwich.' One of the main causes of intestinal wind is swallowed air, either by eating too quickly, or by talking and laughing whilst eating. A common example is slurping your drinks, where air is taken into the stomach which then becomes trapped. The result is great pockets of air which blow you out .

It's hard to train yourself to eat slowly, especially if you were brought up in a household where everyone ate as fast as possible, or if you missed out on second helpings if you ate too slowly. It's hard if you have only a short time in which to eat. The fact is that by eating more slowly and carefully, you will feel full much sooner, and this way you will eat less.

b. Chew your food thoroughly

This goes with eating too quickly. Being in a hurry to finish a meal means that you swallow chunks of food. A typical food-bolter is usually loading the next fork or spoonful before the previous one is swallowed, so train yourself to not return to your plate until your mouth is empty. If you are a die-hard fast eater this will take some discipline, but it has two benefits. Firstly, you will feel satisfied more quickly as the 'full' message takes time to reach the brain. Secondly, you will notice a pleasingly flatter stomach once the air intake is reduced.

c. Try not to eat under stress

Easier said than done, but if a problem is gnawing away at you, or you are sitting at the dinner table fuming after an argument, the effects on your digestion can be pretty unpleasant. The most common complaint is painful stomach cramps an hour or two after eating. An attack of nerves, such as on a first date or before an important interview, can also bring on the most dreadful spasms.

d. Do not leave too long between meals

Leaving long gaps between meals means that we not only get hungry and are therefore more likely to eat more, but the build-up of stomach acid and emptiness can lead to indigestion. Think in terms of this yawning, empty hole in your stomach which suddenly gets a massive amount of food all at once, and probably too quickly. Being on a diet which restricts you to only three meals a day means that you will tend to make the most of every meal. Not only has your stomach been empty for maybe five hours, but it then has to cope with a lot of food in one go. You should not go for more than three hours without something in your stomach if you have a bloating problem.

FLUID RETENTION

The primary cause of bloated stomachs (that feel as if they cannot be held in) is fluid retention. It is nearly always caused by hormones. In a pregnant woman, fluid is retained as a cushion for the growing baby, and in non-pregnant women the reason is similar. Mother Nature's only interest is in the survival of the species, which means that your reproductive organs carry fat and fluid to protect them.

Hormonal activity also encourages you to eat more, and accounts for the sometimes unusual cravings we get when menstruating. Binges occur because the body is craving whatever you are not giving it – notably the enzymes in chocolate. The result of this bingeing is often depression. The high sugar content of chocolate makes your blood sugar level rise sharply. Insulin is activated within the body to counterbalance the raised blood sugar level and unless you eat a significant meal your sugar levels drop dramatically to a very low level. You can feel lacklustre, lethargic, tearful and depressed, and the fact that you've contributed to your weight gain doesn't help.

Years ago, I heard that eating every three hours would banish PMS, from which I used to suffer very badly. All I can say is that I have never looked back. It seems ridiculously simple, but from trying every quack remedy known to man, I went from feeling like a mad woman to not knowing or caring when my next period was.

However, *what* you eat is also important. I stick to my high-starch diet which includes plenty of potatoes, bread and bananas, and I drink a lot of water whether I want to or not. It can be a pain to keep running to the loo, but having a flat stomach with no fluid retention makes it all worthwhile. You need to watch your other foods too, so here's a list which you might find helpful:

1. Foods containing vitamin B

Vitamin B6 has been linked to pre-menstrual syndrome, although in the past people took far too much of it. Over a long period this vitamin can cause loss of sensation and nerve damage in the hands and feet. It is better to obtain vitamin B6 through food, such as:

yeast extract (Marmite), bananas, nuts, cereals, bread, poultry, fish, eggs

An otherwise healthy woman needs only 1.2mg of vitamin B6 a day, which is easily supplied in breakfast cereal or one serving of fish or meat, so a supplement isn't needed.

2. Citrus fruits
Oranges and lemons contain vitamin C which helps the body absorb iron, which helps fight fluid retention.

3. Magnesium-rich foods
Magnesium is also thought to be helpful in the prevention of fluid retention and bloatedness. This is found in:
spinach, nuts, shellfish, dried fruit

4. Vitamin E
Vitamin E is thought to help reduce breast tenderness. It is found in:
olive oil, eggs, wheatgerm, nuts

Finally, do not forget exercise. Exercise is wonderful if you are suffering from cramps, fluid retention and bad moods due to menstruation, both from the point of view of helping your figure, ridding yourself of tension and heightening your mood. Try to take extra *vigorous* exercise at such times, *whether you want to or not*!

PROTEIN DEFICIENCY

It is extremely unlikely to happen in this country, but the swollen stomach condition that we associate with the poverty of Third World countries is due to a total lack of protein in the diet, and is called kwashiorkor. It has occasionally been seen in people who eat mono-diets, such as fruit-only, and is yet another reason to remember that strict crash dieting, or long-term dieting is extremely inadvisable and injurious to the health.

Always eat a good mix of foods. It is what your body wants.

ADDITIVES

We tend to think of additives as causing hyperactivity in children and cancer in laboratory rats. Most of the literature available on additives concentrates, quite rightly, on the defects to our health caused by them. However, purely from the point of view of vanity, I suspect that not many of us are aware of the effects of food additives on our figures.

Additives are thought of as essential because without them

our food would deteriorate more quickly. They prevent hardness and rancidity, and in many cases additives prevent salmonella and other harmful bacteria. It would be wrong to condemn them out of hand, but few people realize that many additives cause the discomfort of abdominal bloating and wind, and the distended stomach we simply can't hold in.

In the quest for a lower-fat diet, manufacturers have had to come up with ever-increasingly weird and wonderful ways of eliminating as many calories as possible from everyday foods, especially high-calorie sweet products and spreads, such as butter, desserts and jams. The result has been the addition of gums, emulsifiers, seaweeds and plain air, in an effort to make it appear that there is more food for fewer calories. The drawbacks have been twofold: you tend to eat twice as much and the additives have unfortunate effects on your digestive system. Why people can't simply eat less of the real thing beats me.

Don't get me wrong. I am not, and never have been additive phobic, nor am I a health freak. I just don't see the point in the tiny calorie saving which usually results from a low-fat alternative if the results are unflattering and embarrassing, as the evidence from dieters bears out.

Here is a list of the most commonly used additives which have a laxative effect, and therefore cause a grumbling and flatulent stomach:

1. Sorbitol – E420, isomalt, mannitol and xylitol

All are artificial sweeteners known to have a laxative effect in high doses. Found in sausages, soft-scoop ice-cream, diabetic jams and sugar-free sweets. In susceptible individuals, especially children, the effects can be a distressingly distended stomach.

2.Carageenan – E407

This seaweed product is an emulsifier, which means that it thickens a product and improves the consistency. Found in quick-setting jellies, milkshakes, biscuits, pastries, meat pies, sausages and instant mousses. Has caused concern for its laxative effect, especially in children.

3. Guar gum (E412), gum arabic (E414) and xanthan gum (E415)

Can cause flatulence through a laxative effect. Found in salad creams, meringue mixes, salad dressings, soft cheese, coleslaw, canned vegetables, processed cheese, pickles, fruit gums, wine, beer, confectionery and yoghurts.

4. Air

Not an additive in the accepted sense, but included here because it is added to some foods to make them appear fuller in volume. An example is ice-cream advertised as low-calorie or low-fat. Taking in extra air is the primary cause of intestinal wind, so avoid foods which boast very low-calorie if possible.

The list of lesser-known and little-used additives which can cause intestinal problems is long, but they need not concern us here as the object is to alert you to the most commonly used additives that you are likely to find in your average foods. I must stress that these substances are not harmful in small doses, but remember that the average diet – especially a slimming diet – will probably include not just one or two, but many of these products every day. The cumulative laxative effect of these additives is something you are unlikely to be aware of. Personally, I see little point in giving up natural sugar and then feeling virtuous by eating large quantities of chemical alternatives instead.

I am not going too deeply into additives as it is not the purpose of this book, but it pays to be aware of the part they play in your goal of a flatter stomach. All my clients who have banished unnecessary additives from their diet and replaced them with fresh and natural foods have always been delighted and astonished at the difference this small change has made to their figures.

You don't want to be chained to the kitchen, but it is so easy to make many of the foods listed above rather than buying them. You'll be glad you made the effort.

IF YOU HAVE A GRUMBLING STOMACH

These remedies are very effective at calming the stomach:
1. Live yoghurt. It contains bacteria which help digestion. On this diet, I have used live yoghurt a great deal, and although it

can be pretty tasteless and bland, the addition of stewed fruit makes it taste really good.

2. Peppermint, fennel and caraway seed teas taken after a meal.

WATER

Water isn't terribly exciting. It is tasteless and makes you run to the loo a lot, which is pretty inconvenient when you're out shopping on a cold winter's day. It's tempting to restrict your fluid intake for a variety of reasons, but try to regard it as not just a physical necessity, but a beauty essential too.

Water is essential in any diet. We need it for digestion and elimination of waste products, and deficiency leads to headaches, constipation and poor concentration. It is also essential to control our body temperature.

Fibre on its own is no good for cleansing the gut. Indeed, when the first fashionable high-fibre diets came on to the market in the 1970s it was common to meet friends who were clutching their stomachs and complaining of severe cramping as the fibre sat in their stomachs, unable to work effectively. Plenty of water should be taken if you eat a lot of insoluble fibre.

You should drink about three pints of water (two litres) a day in the form of either pure water or other drinks such as tea, decaffeinated coffee and pure fruit juices (NOT squash). This is the minimum requirement. What people don't realize is that we get about a third of our fluid intake from our food, and even foods such as meat, poultry and bread contain varying amounts of water. If you are on the sort of diet which is pretty much a starvation regime, and you manage only one meal a day, you are restricting your fluid intake too – hence the well-known 'slimmers' headache' which is caused by dehydration.

Eat plenty of foods which have a high water content. Salad leaves and fruit have as much as 95 per cent water, and most food contains some water.

We do not lose water just through perspiration. Roughly half a pint is lost every day simply through breathing, and another half-pint during our sleep.

If your urine is dark-coloured, strong-smelling and concentrated, you could be at risk from kidney stones. Calcium needs to be diluted otherwise it crystallizes and forms the painful stones. Water flushes out a variety of infections of the bladder as well as waste products.

I do not believe a flatter stomach can be achieved without adequate supplies of drinking water. This should not be the fizzy kind, simply because it has a tendency to increase intestinal wind, but any still water, either bottled or from your tap, can be drunk in abundance. Try to take a positive attitude to drinking water, and accompany every meal with a glass of water. It certainly helps digestion, and the beauty benefits are definitely worth it.

We all hear about dehydrated skins. Part of the problem can be helped with good face creams which help keep moisture in, but one of the causes of wrinkling and puckering of the skin on our faces is lack of fluid. By flushing out waste products and toxins you will also be improving your complexion.

If you are unsure about your domestic water supply, use bottled water. One of my favourite and most refreshing ways to drink water is with slices of fresh orange added. Do try it, it is far nicer than lemon water.

WATER IN OUR FOOD

You may be surprised at the amounts of water in some of our foods:

FRUIT Most fruits are about 70–80 per cent water. Melons contain the most water, at around 90 per cent.

VEGETABLES Most vegetables are nearly 90 per cent water.

BREAD Bread is approximately 38 per cent water.

MEAT AND POULTRY Poultry contains the most water at nearly 70 per cent. Most meats are about 50 per cent water, including sausages.

FISH Most fish contain the same percentage of water, about 75 per cent. Shellfish are about 85 per cent, although smoked fish and anchovies contain less, at around 45 per cent.

CHEESE AND BUTTER Cheese is between 35–55 per cent water, while butter and margarines are about 16 per cent. Very low-fat spreads are about 50 per cent water, which accounts for their low calorie values. Milk is about 90 per cent water.

---

3. YOU SUFFER FROM CONSTIPATION

It may not be a suitable topic of conversation for the dinner table, but the plain fact is that all of us have suffered from constipation at some time or another, and it is undeniably the enemy of elegance.

Modern therapies such as colonic irrigation are a fashionable fad and quite unnecessary. So are purges and laxatives. Long-term use of laxatives can be extremely harmful to your body as they prevent it from functioning in its own natural way and the end result is a lazy gut. They also cause a lot of fluid to be lost from the body which you aren't aware of until you have a blinding headache.

These are the main causes of constipation:
1. Too little fibre and food generally
2. Too little fluid
3. Not enough exercise

In the past few years we have all shovelled down massive quantities of fibre because we are told it is healthy. However, too much fibre on its own is severely irritating to the stomach, and not enough attention has been paid to the fact that it can only work with fluid to ease its passage through the system, so water is essential. Strict dieters are likely to become severely dehydrated because we get a lot of our water from our food (*see the list on page 37*), and the result can be the classic blinding headache and constipation. Our internal plumbing is there for one reason only, and that is to process our food, so too meagre an intake can have serious effects. Lack of exercise, such as in the elderly or the bedridden, has always been known to cause constipation, as any inactivity contributes to the slowing down of the circulation and body functions. Eat regularly, include fibre and take plenty of exercise.

BUT JUST WHAT IS FIBRE?
Fibre is one of two complex carbohydrates. The other is starch.

It may surprise you to know that fibre has no nutritional value and it passes through the large intestine whole, causing a scrubbing action, the results of which are well known to us all. Its old name of roughage was more appropriate to its use, and it is essential for the correct working of the gut. Fibre is also found in vegetables and fruit and some starches which are called 'resistant' because they cannot be digested. However, fibre is an extreme irritant for conditions such as colitis and Irritable Bowel Syndrome, so do take it with caution, or on medical advice.

Insoluble fibre is found in the following:

nuts, rice, bran, strawberries

SOLUBLE FIBRE

There is another type of fibre called 'soluble' which is more easily absorbed by the gut, and which is found in the following foods:

breakfast oats, fruit, vegetables, bread

Dried fruit, wheat bran and whole grains are sources of both types of fibre.

STARCH

Starchy foods used to be unfashionable, especially on diets, as they were thought to be stodgy and fattening. Indeed, as recently as only twenty years ago people were advised to cut down on starches in order to lose weight. We now know that all good diets should contain at least 50 per cent of the daily food intake as starch.

Starchy foods include bread, potatoes, cereals, pasta and rice.

So fibre is a complex carbohydrate. What's a simple carbohydrate?

Simple carbohydrates are sugars:

a) **LACTOSE** from milk and dairy products half as sweet as sugar
b) **GLUCOSE** from vegetables, fruit and honey
c) **SUCROSE** from fruit and vegetables
d) **FRUCTOSE** from fruit and honey
e) **MALTOSE** from malt extract, barley, grains and malted wheat

A high-carbohydrate diet replenishes and increases the body's reserve of glycogens, which are especially important in giving you energy and making you feel lively. A common complaint of dieters over the years has been the tiredness that almost always used to accompany low-calorie diets, but by eating the correct balance of proteins, carbohydrates and fats you should be able to lose weight steadily, and with no ill-effects.

4. YOUR MUSCLES NEED TONING

If you want to succeed, you must exercise. I have already said that obsessive exercise for the sake of eating an extra slice of pizza is stressful and unnecessary, but the secret of lasting slimness continues to include regular exercise. Exercise increases your resting metabolism, so that calories are being burned at a faster rate even when you are doing nothing. Exercise increases your circulation which brings beauty benefits too. Never give up on exercise. The days of pumping iron and sweating on a treadmill may be over for some but having said that, I know that many women still enjoy their aerobics classes and gym sessions for the social side as well, and I'm all for that. Speaking as someone who has taken many thousands of exercise classes, I also know that the symptoms of the menopause and PMS are greatly relieved by more strenuous exercise, so if that is the way you like to look after yourself, do continue.

DOING IT THE NATURAL WAY

We don't realize just how well our stomach muscles can be exercised in the natural way, by walking, going up and down stairs, gardening and cycling. There's no need to ever go to a sports club, and indeed many people live miles from the nearest leisure facility so have little choice but to go it alone. I couldn't drive a car until I was in my thirties, so walking or cycling were the only means of getting about, and I'm glad. These days we start up the car and take the children to school at the slightest hint of rain; people cycle only when it's dry. We weren't meant to spend our lives sitting on our bottoms, and the sedentary life is far more to blame for weight problems than what we eat. Frankly, we could eat anything we wanted if we walked a couple of miles a day.

Swimming is wonderful for toning the muscles, and the stretching action is marvellous for our posture. All types of sweeping work, hoovering the carpet or raking leaves will tone up your muscles if you remember to pull in your abdomen as you sweep, to prevent all the effort being taken by your back. Your abdominal muscles simply act as a corset, and help the action of your back.

WHICH EXERCISE?

It's always assumed that if people just take more exercise their figure problems will go away. Indeed, increasing exercise, while undoubtedly making you lose weight, will not tone up specific areas of your body. It is different types of exercise *combined* which are the key to a lovely figure. For example, I know of several women who needed to lose weight and started step aerobics, only to find that they lost weight but developed enormous legs! Or others who have gone cycling in order to develop their calves, which is entirely the wrong type of exercise. You need the right exercise for your own needs and right now, we want a flatter stomach.

If you are a complete beginner, if you have health problems, bad knees and have never done more than walk to the kitchen, you won't want to wade straight in with 100 sit-ups before breakfast. Neither will you welcome my suggestion of a gentle morning stroll if you've just completed the London Marathon. I leave it to you to decide which options to go for in my list of exercise ideas. The main thing to do, though, is to *increase* whatever you are doing now, and to do *more* floor exercises every day. So if you are doing nothing in the way of exercise, it's best to start with about five minutes of warm-up and stomach-tightening exercises, adding some extra aerobic exercise every day. If you are a hot-shot expert, go the whole hog with advanced abdominal exercises five times a day, and an extra forty-five minutes of aerobic work such as swimming or cycling. Whatever you are doing, do more of it!

It's as well to take a moment to explain the difference between different types of exercise and training categories:
1. Strength 2. Flexibility 3. Aerobic

5 D A Y S T O A F L A T T E R S T O M A C H

It is important to understand how each component contributes to achieving any figure goal.

EXERCISE FOR MUSCLE STRENGTH AND TONE

This doesn't mean you're training to be a weightlifter. Giving your muscles tone means they get stronger and look better, but you won't be in any way muscle bound unless you start to use heavy weights. In any case, a woman's body composition is such that we are unlikely to get as muscular as a man. Strength and toning exercise will tone your muscles but won't specifically help you lose weight.

We all know what muscle looks like if we've ever cut up a piece of meat. Lean meat is the muscle of the animal, and it has fibres running through it. What makes the difference between each of us is the number of fibres in our muscles, which depends on how much we use them.

It is possible to have almost no muscle at all. If you are starving, your body will consume anything it can to stay alive, and the result is tremendous weakness. In fact, the body consumes muscles *before* fat in a situation of extreme food deprivation such as anorexia or crash diets, but that is a subject which whole books have been written on, and all we need to know is that when we exercise, a slice of fat doesn't magically disappear from the top of each thigh!

SO WHAT WILL STRENGTH TRAINING DO, AND WHAT WON'T IT DO?

1. It will NOT improve flexibility
2. It WILL tone and tighten your muscles
3. It will only SLIGHTLY improve aerobic capacity

FLEXIBILITY EXERCISE

You can't look good if you don't stretch. Modern ways of exercising have left women with bowed, muscular thighs, thick ankles and large calves. Many women would call themselves fit, yet they can't straighten their knees. Nor can they press a hand into the space between their shoulder blades or touch their toes. They might have a body–fat ratio to die for, but total fitness includes muscles which can operate over a large range and that means they should be flexible and easily stretched to avoid injury. An individual who is fit but not flexible cannot be said to have all-round fitness.

Beauty is an entire effect. Some people train themselves into the ground for the body beautiful, then shower and slouch off with their sports bag weighing down their shoulders. No thought of elegance. No line to the body or beauty of movement. No point.

Flexibility training should be included as part of your daily activities from now on. A flat stomach depends on having a nice line to your body with long, lean and stretched muscles. By lifting your ribcage and lengthening your abdominal muscles which are well stretched, you can improve the appearance of your stomach by several inches.

During this plan, I want you to warm up, mobilize your joints and stretch out every morning.

AEROBIC EXERCISE AND THE FAT-BURNING ISSUE

Unfortunately some exercise experts have been allowed to get away with murder in recent years. I watched a video recently where the presenter, a Hollywood actress, said after about fifteen minutes of warm-up, '. . . now we're going to really start to burn some fat!'. This is misleading. If fat burning was so easy, our hips and thighs would be going in and out like yo-yos as we put on the fat, then went out to an aerobics class and *hey presto!* it would vanish. Our systems simply don't work like that.

We have come to think of aerobics as meaning aerobics *classes*. In fact, the term simply means 'with air' and in the scientific world the term has been used for years to describe the form of metabolism involving energy liberated in a muscle in the presence of oxygen. Aerobic activities include brisk walking, running, cycling and swimming – in fact any activity which increases your heart rate, gets your blood pumping harder and which makes you feel a bit breathless. It does *not* burn fat as such, or at least it will not do so until you have been exercising for some considerable time. The best way to rid yourself of fat by using it as fuel is to increase the rate at which your body uses its energy, and we do that by raising our metabolic rates.

It is not sensible to constantly look at food intake and exercise as a credit and debit situation. You shouldn't think of it as being all right to have a chocolate eclair as long as you can go swimming and use up the extra calories. Once your metabolic system is up and running you can take several special meals or a holiday or a heavy weekend in your stride. Your body has its own natural weight and will continually strive to stay there. Think in terms of averaging out your food intake and increasing your metabolic rate with more daily exercise.

Muscle is different from fat, and muscle doesn't run to fat, as used to be thought the case. Muscle is one thing and fat another, but the difference is that muscle is alive while fat just sits there as your emergency fuel supplies. Muscle has its own blood supply which is serviced by the oxygen you breathe, and muscle works hard and gets hot when you are exercising. Fat doesn't do anything, except sit and wobble! It's true that if you exercise for long enough your fat stores will kick in to supply you with the missing energy, but it takes a long time for that to happen, and you'll probably have gone home by then. So if you weigh nine stone, is it nine stone of fat or muscle?

Eating, digesting and absorbing food will increase your metabolism, simply because it is another job for your body to do. Starvation diets, or restrictive diets which allow you only a couple of meals a day and no in-between snacks actually *lower* your metabolic rate because the fall in your blood glucose levels leads to your body switching in to its survival mechanism of energy conservation. If you become so thin that your lean muscle tissue also decreases – as in the case of anorexia – your resting metabolic rate goes so low that it is completely counter-productive in weight loss. You also put weight back on extremely quickly after such a regime, and often by eating very little.

A QUICK CALORIE COUNT

I don't approve of counting calories for the sake of it, but just for fun, and to cheer you up if you are stuck in an office or at home and can't get out much, here is a list of the calories spent doing a variety of ordinary chores:

SLEEPING	30	SWEEPING	90
MAKING BEDS	120	TYPING	60
STANDING STILL	45	DRIVING	60
EATING	45	MOWING LAWN	225
WASHING DISHES	60	DIGGING GARDEN	240
WASHING CLOTHES	90	MODERATE CYCLING	120
WRITING	60	RACING CYCLING	330
IRONING	60	SQUASH	420
KNITTING	45	AEROBICS	200–300
MOPPING FLOOR	120	BRISK WALKING	180

EXERCISING AT HOME

If you're unable to get out of the house, or there aren't any decent facilities near you or you haven't got transport, don't worry. When my children were small I was in the same position and still managed a 'daily dozen' in my own living-room just three times a day when the children were either having a nap or playing. Sometimes they even joined me in jigging about to some music. Here is a typical exercise routine:

ALWAYS WARM UP

The purpose of a warm-up is to prepare the body for exercise. Muscles which are cold – and remember that even on the hottest day your muscles will not be ready for action if they have been at rest – will not stretch, and will tear easily.

A proper warm-up is important for these reasons:
1. It increases blood flow
2. Mobilizes the joints
3. Raises heart rate
4. Prepares the body for exercise

If you are particularly inactive, overweight or over seventy, this warm-up should be done every day, regardless of whether you continue on with further exercise.

5 DAYS TO A FLATTER STOMACH

Warm-up exercises

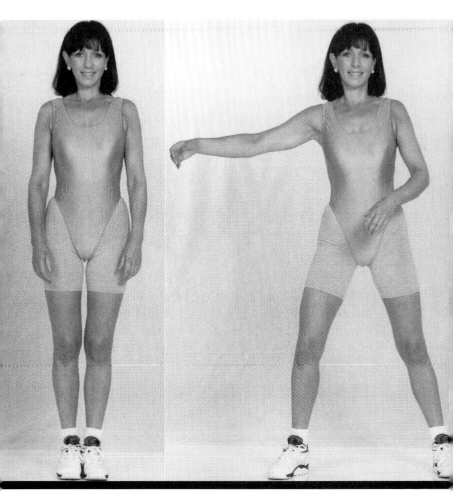

Side steps and arm swings
Simply step from side to side, swinging your arms.
Swing gently at first, then higher.

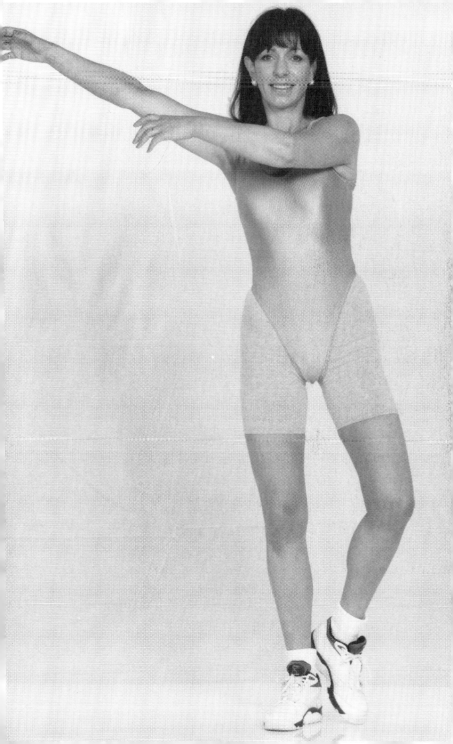

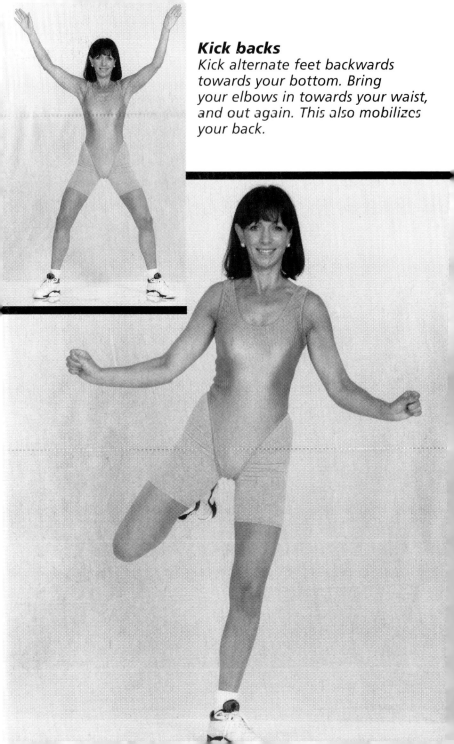

Kick backs
Kick alternate feet backwards towards your bottom. Bring your elbows in towards your waist, and out again. This also mobilizes your back.

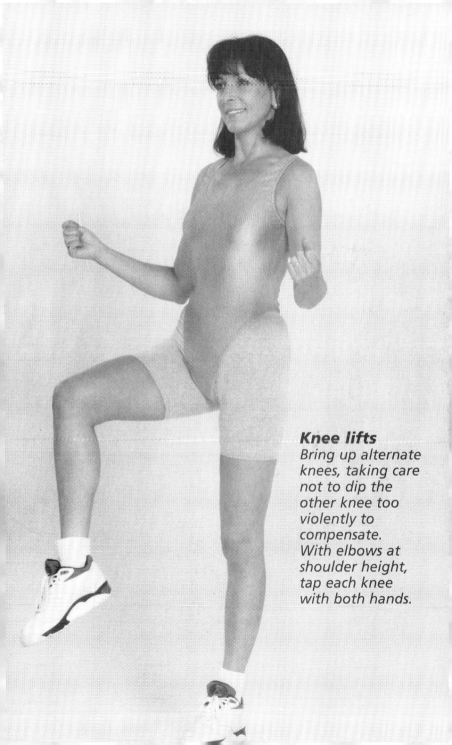

Knee lifts

Bring up alternate knees, taking care not to dip the other knee too violently to compensate. With elbows at shoulder height, tap each knee with both hands.

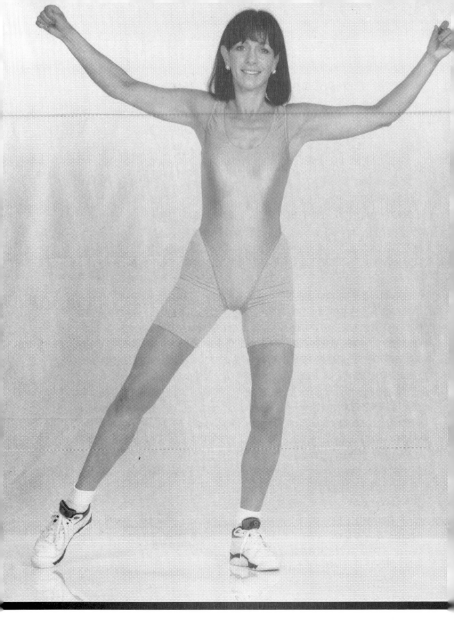

Half-jacks

Starting with feet together, stretch each leg to side.
Arms raise to sides and down again. Change legs.

Mobilizing your joints

If you think about it, most of us go through our lives never putting our joints through their full range of movement. Think for example of these joints, and their capabilities:

1. The Knee
Capable of movement in one direction only. Put it through its range of motion daily, by bringing the foot backwards towards your bottom, and holding it there for about ten seconds. Do this after your warm-up.

2. The Shoulder
Your shoulder is the only joint which is capable of movement in a complete circle, yet how many times in the average week or month do you make your shoulder do all that it is capable of? Do six to ten complete shoulder circles each side, every day.

3. The Hip
The hip is another joint which gets badly neglected by sedentary people, and even those who take a lot of exercise. Easily mobilized through swimming the breast-stroke, at home you can do simple leg-hugs.

4. The Wrists and Ankles
On the whole, I am of the opinion that if you can move around, put on your make-up, comb your hair and walk well, your wrists and ankles get quite sufficient mobilization during general use.

However, don't forget to circle your ankles and wrists every day, especially if you do work such as typing or sitting still a lot, just to keep stiffness at bay.

Stretching out

The following stretches are standard, and should be done after your warm-up and before aerobic exercise. Repeat at the end of your workout:

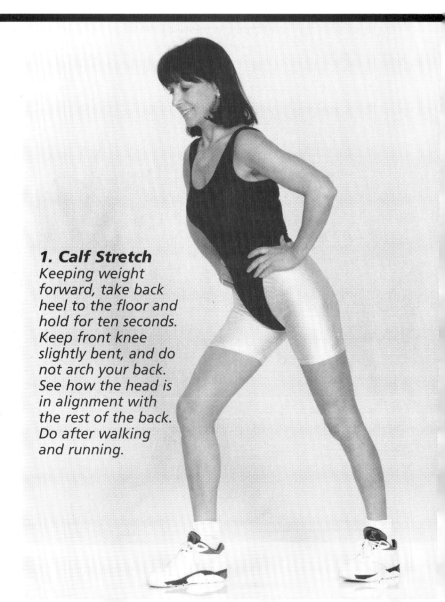

1. Calf Stretch
Keeping weight forward, take back heel to the floor and hold for ten seconds. Keep front knee slightly bent, and do not arch your back. See how the head is in alignment with the rest of the back. Do after walking and running.

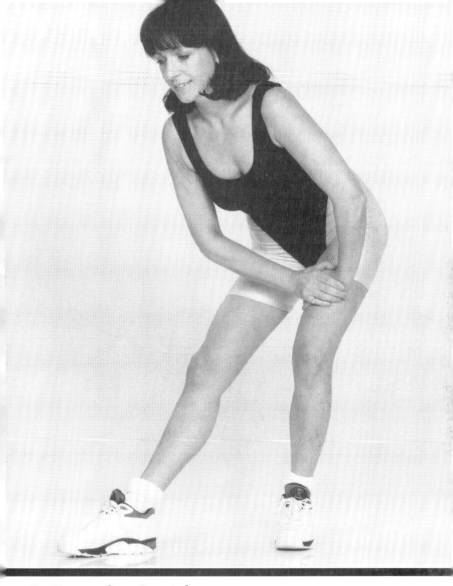

2. Hamstring Stretch

Bend the left knee. Resting both hands on the left thigh (not your knee), stretch the right leg forwards, foot flat to floor. Lean slightly forwards. Hold for ten seconds. Change legs.

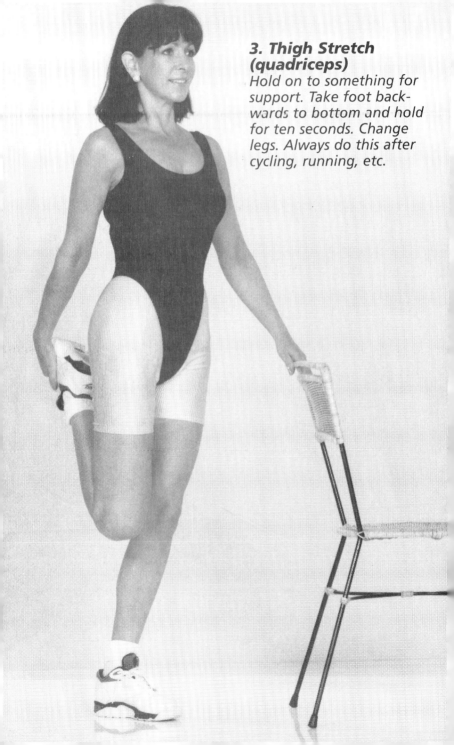

3. Thigh Stretch (quadriceps)

Hold on to something for support. Take foot backwards to bottom and hold for ten seconds. Change legs. Always do this after cycling, running, etc.

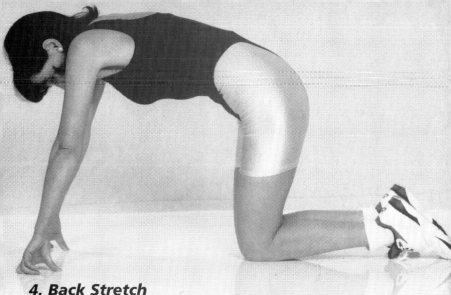

4. Back Stretch

On all fours, do a 'cat stretch' by arching then dipping your back. Do four of each.

5. Chest Stretch (pectoral)

Important for good posture (p. 66). Place palms of hands in the small of your back, press inwards and draw shoulder blades together. Drop head slightly. Hold for ten seconds, release and repeat three more times.

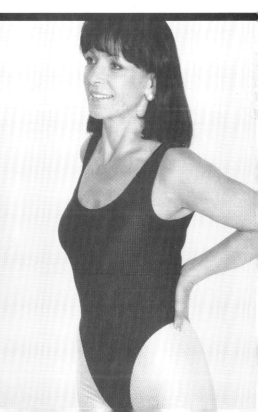

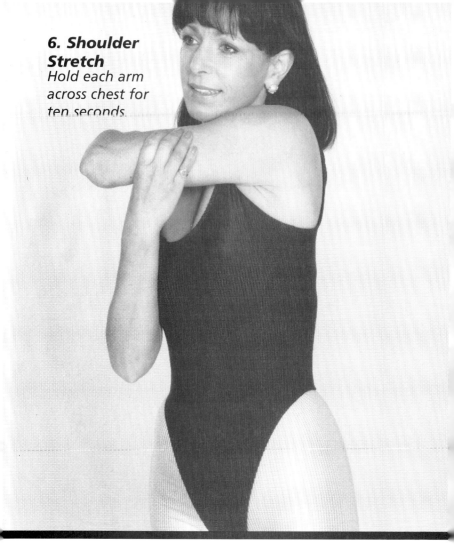

6. Shoulder Stretch
Hold each arm across chest for ten seconds.

These are the main stretches which you must do every day. There are many more other stretches which you might add to this repertoire if you are engaged in a particularly demanding workout routine, but the average woman who cares enough about her figure should make this routine as much a part of her day as doing her hair.

This warm up, mobilization and stretch routine should be done every morning. It takes about five minutes.

Your 5 abdominal exercises

I am going to give you just 5 variations on the standard stomach strengthening exercise. They are:

1. The Foundation
2. The Crunch
3. The Waist Whittler
4. The Chair lift
5. The Air Bike

It is important that you understand that you *do not have to do* all the variations. If you are new to abdominal exercise, if you have been ill or have had a baby, it is best just to stay with The Foundation exercise until you are stronger. It will be quite enough to keep you toned and trim, and as you progress, add in The Waist Whittler which is another quite basic exercise. If you are already accustomed to exercise, I suggest you do all five exercises between three and five times a day.

A WORD OF WARNING
Always be sure that you have warmed up first, and that you are wearing loose clothing.

THE FOUNDATION

Abdominal exercises are not always easy to get right. People complain that their necks ache and their backs hurt. If anything ever hurts, *stop at once*. There can be several reasons for the pain:

1. Your position is wrong
2. You have done too many repetitions
3. You are tired
4. It is the wrong time of the month

Number four is important because your monthly cycle can affect the way you exercise to quite a marked degree. In the week or so before your period, hormones are pouring into your body which mimic pregnancy in a small way, and your ligaments can be a little vulnerable. Women often suffer from minor injuries, which they wouldn't normally experience around this time, so take care. It doesn't mean you shouldn't exercise however.

1. Start off with your feet flat on the floor, about hip-width apart.

2. Place both hands right under the bulge at the back of your head. Look at the ceiling.

3. Lift your head, but let your hands take its weight.

4. Make your chest and your head and neck one piece, in one line. The best way to think of your upper position is that the line of your top half should not be broken by the hinge of the neck.

*5. Inhale before you start. Exhale, and **press your stomach downwards**. Tilt your pelvis up towards your chest and neck. Lift without breaking the line by tugging on your head or jerking it upwards. Press downwards.*
This pattern of breathing should continue throughout. You breathe *in* before you start, or on the release of effort. You

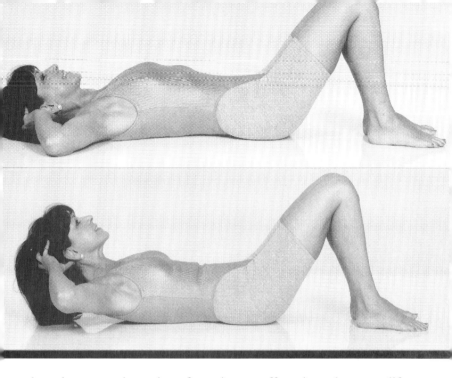

breathe *out* at the point of maximum effort, i.e. when you lift
and press downwards.

*6. Good! Now you have mastered the form of the sit-
up, do eight, slowly.*

7. Do eight more repetitions.

*8. Have a rest for ten seconds, bring your knees into
your chest.*

*9. Repeat the exercise, doing eight or sixteen
repetitions, according to how you feel.*

*10. Stretch out by turning over and lifting yourself on
to your elbows.*

THE CRUNCH

1. This time, lift your feet off the floor and cross your ankles. Feel the small of your back pressed firmly to the floor.

*2. Take your upper position, as for The Foundation, neck and chest in one line. Support your head with your hands behind your head. As before, do **not** pull on your neck. Your head and back should be in **one line**.*

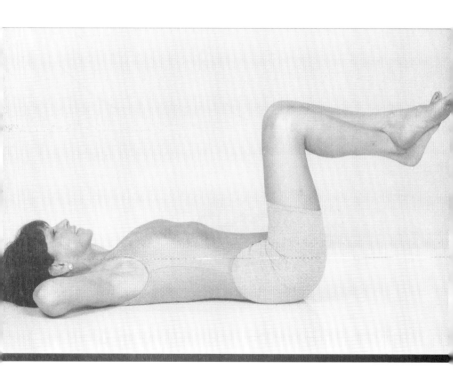

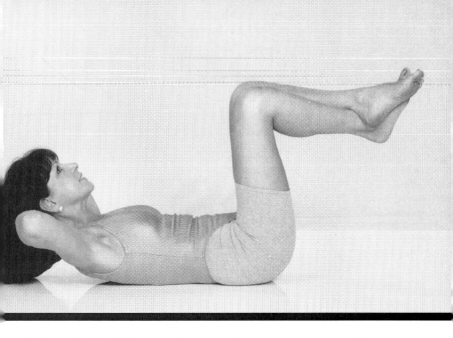

3. Breathe in, lift your chest and press your stomach **downwards**, exhaling as you do so. Do four, up and down, slowly, then do eight double-time pulses, then repeat the four slow crunches.

4. Turn over and stretch out to decompress your spine.

THE WAIST WHITTLER

Without this exercise, your oblique muscles, which lie around your ribcage area and which shape your waist, sit there, do nothing and are slack. This exercise does not increase the number of muscle fibres because you are not using weight. It tones and stretches the muscles so they become taut, and give you a tighter, smaller waist.

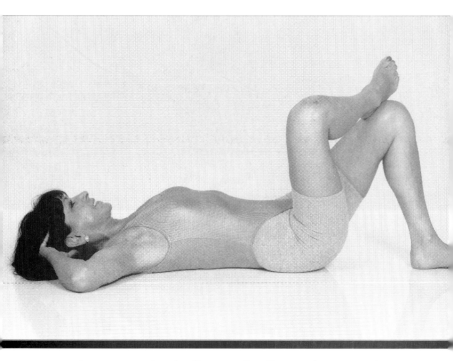

1. Lie on your back, flat on the floor. Place one foot on floor, the other across the other thigh. Both hands support your head at the nape of your neck. Look at the ceiling. Breathe in.

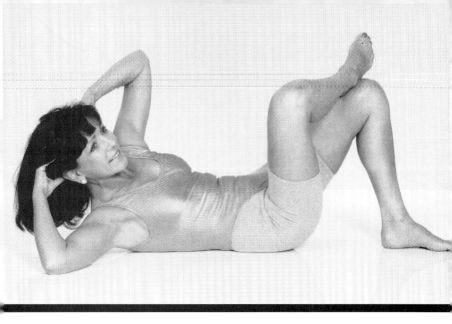

*2. Breathe out and reach left shoulder across to the right knee. If you find this hard to do, don't worry because it isn't important to **reach** the other knee. You must let your head **fall back** into your hand and keep looking up towards the ceiling. **Don't tug your neck**. Breathe in again as you release back to the floor.*

3. Do eight, change sides, repeat the eight.

*4. Turn over and decompress your spine by raising on to your elbows. Remember to keep your head and neck in alignment with your spine by looking **down** at the floor.*

THE CHAIR LIFT

This exercise is slightly easier if you find it hard to keep your legs up. It also stops your legs from helping you, thereby giving your stomach muscles all the hard work!

1. Lie on floor with your bottom about 18in from the base of a chair. Place your legs from the knee downwards on the chair. Cross your arms behind your head.

2. Breathe in first. Breathe out, and press downwards with your abdomen, raising your upper body as you do so. You won't come up very high.

3. Lower and breathe in, expanding your chest as you do so. Repeat eight times, rest and repeat a further eight.

4. Turn over and decompress your spine.

5. Return to starting position and repeat the two sets of eight. Decompress.

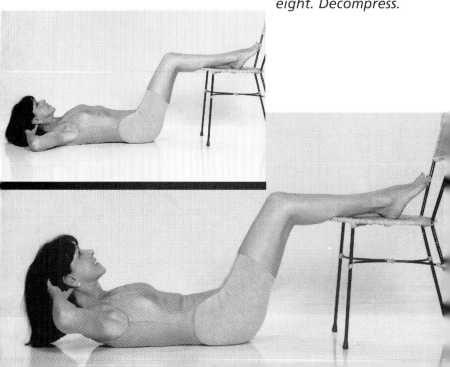

THE AIR BIKE

Only do this exercise if you are NOT severely overweight, and if you can be sure to keep your legs up in the air. It isn't a failing if you find it hard – you'll work up to it soon enough!

Take position as in picture
The exercise should be self-explanatory. What you must NOT do, however, is simply swivel your elbows wildly fromside to side.

Pulse slowly up to each knee as it comes in towards your face, then stretching out the leg towards the ceiling. Do eight or sixteen slowly, *according to your level of fitness and strength.* Rest, repeat the set then turn over to stretch out.

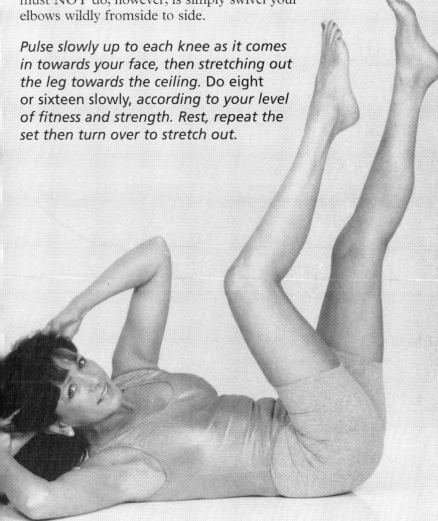

5. YOUR POSTURE IS TERRIBLE

There's no point in losing weight if you're going to ruin the effect by slouching. Exercising your body to perfection, dieting yourself into the ground and spending a fortune on clothes is time and money wasted if your chest droops, your neck caves in and your stomach sticks out – all because you don't stand properly.

Good posture is best judged when it is lacking. Not only is it vital to the beauty of your figure, but it has effects on your digestion, breathing and general health, including your back. Bad posture places strain on ligaments and muscles leading to pain, stiffness and general lack of mobility.

Nearly everything we do pulls us inwards and downwards contributing to poor posture. We are designed to face one way and all our movements lead in that direction – inwards and downwards. We bend down to pick things up, we lean forwards to write, type and eat. We have no occasion to lean backwards, or to carry out a task with our hands behind our backs. We were meant to live on all fours.

I was standing at the supermarket checkout the other day, behind a woman who had a trim bottom encased in skin-tight jeans, a snug T-shirt and who held great promise of being just as gorgeous from the front. Finally she turned round and my jaw nearly dropped open, because she had a particularly prominent stomach. It wasn't just your average little bulge, and she clearly wasn't pregnant. Her chest slouched down to her navel, her bust hung unattractively and her stomach protruded. And this was all down to posture.

Good posture is a habit. One of the worst things you can do is to stand for a long time, yet this might be part of your work. The natural tendency when standing is to lean backwards, but this conjures up pictures of slanting bodies which look as if they are compensating for a stiff breeze. What we do is stick our hips forwards and balance the top half of our bodies on top of the pelvis, so the socket joints of our hips are taking all the strain of the pelvis. Do it, and you'll see what I mean. This in turn has the effect of thrusting the abdomen forwards and there you have your sticking-out stomach. It takes a conscious effort to pull yourself back into alignment, and we need constant reminders. If you are not used to it, standing properly feels awkward and wrong. Your lower back muscles are used to taking all the strain and your stomach muscles are used to doing nothing, so the first exercise is to train your stomach muscles to hold you in a straighter line, thereby taking the effort away from your back. Below is the typical backwards lean of the body at rest. It causes what is known as 'kyphosis':

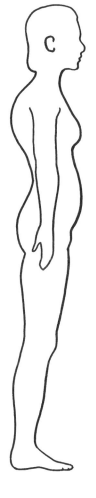

KYPHOSIS

Rounded shoulders are often the result of tight chest muscles, which are caused either by a particular working practice or by over-development of the pectoral muscles through weight training or sports. Tight chest muscles cause the chest to become concave and the shoulders to round forwards.

Note the effect on the abdomen

The best way to correct this fault is to stretch the pectoral (chest) muscles every day, and to strengthen the spinal muscles in the chest. An added bonus is an improved bustline.

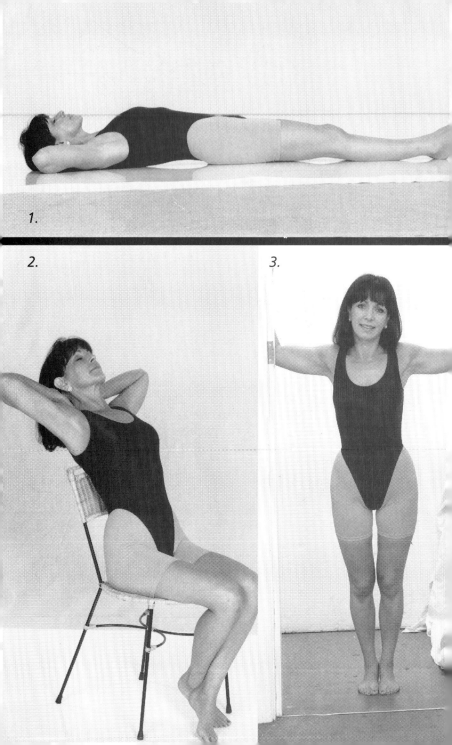

1.

2.

3.

Pectoral stretches

1. Lie flat on floor. Place flat palms under your head, and press elbows to the floor. Hold for ten seconds, rest for ten seconds, and repeat five times.

2. Another way to stretch the pectoral muscles is by leaning backwards in a chair, in which the back of the chair only comes as far as the shoulder blades. Place the hands behind the neck. Press inwards with the palms and outwards with the elbows.

3. Another good exercise to try every day helps a sagging abdomen by training you to lift upwards and outwards from your ribcage.
Stand in a doorway. Pressing the arms against the sides of the doorway, raise up on to the toes and lean forwards very slightly. Keep the stretch for ten seconds, rest and repeat.

When you have finished these stretches, stand in front of a full-length mirror and see the improvement in your posture.

All these exercises promote strengthening of the upper back and chest muscles, leading to an improvement in the appearance of the trunk, an uplift to the bustline and a consequent decrease in the perceived size of the abdomen.

These exercises should be practised every day on waking, in the middle of the day and in the evening, until they become second nature.

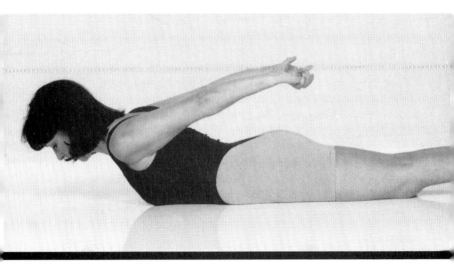

Rounded shoulders may be due to shortened and tight pectoral muscles or to weak muscles in the upper back (the rhomboid and trapezius muscles). This exercise strengthens those muscles.

Lie on your stomach. Clasp your hands behind your back and gently raise the shoulders and chest off the floor.

Another common fault of people who sit at a desk, telephone or work station all day, and especially people who do a lot of driving is this:

THE DOWAGER'S HUMP

This postural fault is caused by a poor sitting position over a period of time, common in office workers. The chin juts forward and the upper spine curves to compensate. The abdominal muscles are unable to work properly and the pelvis tips backwards, resulting in a sagging appearance. Note that the figure illustrated is not overweight, yet the stomach appears large and unsightly.

Apart from your hairstyle and weight, nothing is more ageing than poor posture. Rightly or wrongly we associate stooped figures with old people, and next time you see someone who seems young for their age, make a note of what it is about them that makes them appear this way. It is not just good skin or hair or slimness. A sprightly step and a good carriage are what mark people out as looking younger. A sagging stomach suggests neglect, fatigue and a generally lacklustre attitude to life. We've all seen women in their twenties looking like this. Standing properly lifts your ribcage and flattens your stomach.

Get into the habit of practising your posture in front of a full-length mirror every morning. It will soon become second nature.

THESE ARE YOUR FIVE POSTURE EXERCISES WHICH YOU MUST REMEMBER TO DO EVERY DAY.

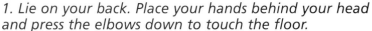

1. Lie on your back. Place your hands behind your head and press the elbows down to touch the floor.
2. Sit in a chair and lean backwards. Place the hands behind the neck, press out with your elbows.
3. Stand in a doorway. Press the arms into the sides of the doorway, raise yourself on to your toes and lean forwards slightly. Hold for ten seconds.
4. Lie on your stomach. Clasp the hands behind the back and raise the shoulders and chest off the floor. This stretches your chest.
5. Stand with a book on your head. Feel the neck lengthening and the jaw slightly tilting forwards. Lift the chest. Hold for ten seconds, then slowly walk round the room.

Wearing the right clothes

Clothes can make a lot of difference to how our bodies are perceived, and if you are rarely satisfied when you study yourself in the mirror, especially when you have just spent a couple of hours trying things on and discarding them, maybe now's the time to ask yourself if you should be trying something else.

The same goes for clothes which are unflattering on our stomachs. If you are tall you're going to have a head-start on all of us shorter women. The sheer body length stretches everything and gives a greater impression of slimness. However, if you do have a weight problem and particularly a big stomach problem, it's better not to wear clothes which cinch you in at the waist, leaving your midriff spilling out over the top and your lower stomach bulging out breathlessly from underneath.

Making the most of your figure means just that, and it pays to emphasize your good bits. Everyone has something they don't worry about, so find yours. If you have good legs but your figure goes haywire in the middle, shift dresses are the best type to wear, or short, boxy jackets which skim your waist but don't hug your hips.

The general theory of corsets, girdles and all-in-ones was that they stopped you using your stomach muscles. I don't agree. They certainly make you stand up straight, and with an artificially flat stomach you can wear all sorts of clinging little numbers you'd never dream of wearing if your body was free range.

Do give your clothes a thought. A tight skirt or pair of trousers are often your only benchmark to the state you're in, and plenty of women have told me they never weigh themselves, but go by the fit of a particular item of clothing. Your posture and the way you hold in your stomach are vital elements in a flatter stomach, and wearing forgiving items of clothing does nothing to aid this process. Get rid of stretchy leggings, elastic-waisted skirts and tracksuit bottoms. Looking sloppy means that all your hard work is completely undone.

2

The Diet

....

So what am I going to eat?

*D*oes starting a new diet mean your house begins to look like a Harvest Festival? Do you have to spend the first morning scurrying between shops for all those ritzy herbs and vegetables your diet magazine told you to get? Maybe you need a day's holiday just to sort out who's eating what as you juggle one meal for yourself, another for the toddler and something else for when your mother-in-law visits?

Surely this preoccupation with food is what got us into this mess in the first place? Learning about tasty, delicious and inventive ways with food isn't my idea of cutting down and losing weight, so save your gourmet recipes either for your off-diet days or for when you've reached your goal and can trust yourself. On this diet everything is plain, simple food which everyone likes, and nothing takes long to make, so stay out of the kitchen, or spend as little time as possible in it, at least for the next five days.

Although my golden rule is that food should be simple and plain while on a diet plan, this doesn't mean boring. Smoked salmon, soufflés and herb omelettes are simple, but chic. Plain food is wonderful for your figure. So batten down the hatches for a few days and stock up on starch. This is a **proper** diet.

The rules

In order for this diet to work and for you to lose weight and get a flatter stomach, it is vital that you keep to these golden rules:

1. Eat every three hours
2. Stick to starch during the day
3. NO fruit during the day, except bananas
4. NO bran or insoluble fibre (peas, sweetcorn, etc.) in day
5. Stick to the portion control rules – NOTHING is unlimited
6. NO artificial sweeteners, low-fat or low-calorie products
7. Drink water with every meal, and between meals
8. Have a high-fibre snack during the evening
9. NEVER skip breakfast even if you are not hungry
10. NEVER go to bed empty

IN ADDITION, THESE ARE YOUR GUIDELINES FOR EATING

1. Don't put more on your plate than your portion allowances. You can always go back for more
2. Don't load the next fork or spoonful before the previous mouthful has been swallowed
3. If you feel full, stop at once. Put the plate aside and come back to it later
4. Don't swallow your food until it is thoroughly chewed
5. Where possible, as in the case of apples, slice food up first rather than eat it whole. This encourages moderation

I apologize if this sounds like a mother teaching her children table manners, but problems with food and weight often have their root cause in bad eating habits. Don't treat every meal as if you won't get the chance to eat it ever again.

YOUR 5-DAY SHOPPING LIST

(This list covers all of the alternatives, but remember you only need to make the dishes you like, so you won't need everything from this list):

1. VEGETABLES – potatoes, carrots, French beans, carrots, tinned and baby sweetcorn, red, green and yellow peppers, avocado, tinned chopped tomatoes, onions, broccoli, garlic, peas, mushrooms, green salad, aubergine, celery, mange-touts, bean sprouts, red and white cabbage

2. RICE – long-grain, basmati, short-grain (pudding)

3. PASTA – spirals, fusilli, spaghetti

4. BREAD – preferably white unbleached, though you will also need some wholemeal, muffins or crumpets

5. FRUIT – apples, bananas, grapes, strawberries, lemon, grape-fruit, sultanas or raisins, blackberries, pear, dried fruit

6. FISH – salmon or cod, smoked salmon, smoked mackerel, tinned sardines, plaice

7. MEAT – chicken breasts (skinless and boneless), lean minced beef, lamb chops

8. CEREAL – Shredded Wheat, Weetabix or bran flakes, porridge oats (or Rice Crispies if you need gluten-free cereal)

10. DAIRY – live bio-yoghurt, butter, skimmed milk, eggs, Cheddar cheese, *crème fraîche*, cottage cheese

11. DRESSINGS AND SAUCES – vinaigrette dressing (see p.157), mayonnaise (see p.157), chilli sauce, golden syrup, jam, gravy, mint sauce, pesto sauce, white wine vinegar

12. TINNED TOMATO PASTE OR PURÉE

13. HERBS AND SPICES – fresh or dried tarragon, dill, basil, oregano, salt and freshly ground black pepper, mustard powder, parsley, chilli, ginger paste, garlic purée, turmeric, nutmeg, cinnamon stick, cloves, Oxo cube

14. OIL – olive, corn, walnut, hazelnut

15. NUTS AND SEEDS – Brazil nuts, almonds, walnuts, sunflower seeds

16. PULSES – tinned chickpeas

17. DRINKS – mineral water, tea, decaffeinated coffee, apple juice

You do not have to go out and buy expensive foods like salmon and prawns if you don't wish to. You might not have a kitchen which is up to a lot of preparation and cooking, or you might live on your own and find making a whole dish just too compli-cated and time-consuming. However, the diet lasts only five days and is intended to produce results, so it's worth putting yourself out to get the right foods.

I have included a vegetarian recipe section and most of the pasta dishes are suitable for vegetarians, but I generally find that most vegetarians are expert at adapting ideas for their own tastes.

CALORIE COUNTING

On the whole, I am not in favour of calorie obsession. It is sufficient to know that with our very small portions your daily content will be enough for you to lose weight, but I have included calories in the recipe section simply because I thought you might be surprised at how low-calorie some of the meals are, especially as they contain ingredients such as cream and cheese.

WHAT WILL I DRINK?

Sorry to be a party pooper. No alcohol is allowed on the standard five-day plan, but it won't kill you. When you progress to The Maintenance Plan, you can have a couple of glasses of wine a day, lager or the odd glass of champagne, if you choose.

Every meal must be accompanied by a glass of water, and leave a glass handy so you can sip it whenever you walk past. I keep a glass of still mineral water on my desk with a straw in it, so I can have a quick sip every now and again. When water only came from a tap, asking for it at parties and in pubs attracted comment – now that it comes in coloured bottles and costs a fortune it's suddenly fashionable. Try adding a slice of orange or lemon, for variety.

In addition, drink tea and decaffeinated coffee as you wish. NO fizzy drinks are allowed as they have a tendency to make you feel full and bloated.

WHAT IF I GET HUNGRY?

Never go hungry. A starchy snack does you no harm, and if it keeps you from the biscuit tin, all the better. There's nothing worse than a diet which only allows three meals a day, as it encourages diet breaking and bingeing if you're sitting looking at the clock with your tummy rumbling and a headache coming on. I would be surprised if you felt hungry while you follow this plan but if you are, have one of the following:

A slice of bread or toast
Some cold potatoes
A couple of spoonfuls of Rice Crispies with skimmed milk
A banana

If you can, however, try to be positive and realize that you don't get anything for nothing. A flatter stomach is a prize worth having, and constant gratification every time your tummy rumbles means weight gain, so get used to the discipline of your meal times. It will take some getting used to, which is why you are allowed a snack, but the objective is to realign your eating habits and the way you think about eating and hunger. Accept hunger, but don't be afraid of eating.

THE RECIPES

We're back to discipline being liberating. It's like those restaurant menus which go on forever and take half an hour to decipher – I prefer about three choices, then I can get on with enjoying the company instead of dithering. Wondering what to have for supper can be surprisingly stressful, so I have restricted the recipes to a sensible number which you might reasonably get through on this diet. I have chosen them for the speed of preparation, ease of buying and relative low cost. They were all mentioned by my testers as particular favourites.

CHOPPING AND CHANGING THE MEALS

I would prefer it if you ate a decent lunch and a smaller evening meal, which is how I like to eat, as I believe it is the secret of successful slimming. However, as the majority of the population prefers to dine in the evening I have aimed the larger meal for that time of day. Feel free to swap about and if you have a particularly late meal, you might want to bring your supper forwards. As long as you stay with the three-hour rule, there's no point in turning your life upside down!

HOW ABOUT CONVENIENCE FOODS?

I know that it's easier to buy a tray of something which you can microwave, but if you read the list of ingredients, even the simplest sounding ready meal contains some real horrors. As I said in the additives section, there's nothing wrong or dangerous about any of these additives, except in quantity, but so many of them are irritating or laxative for the stomach and remember, this is a flat stomach plan.

Making a plate of mashed potatoes, or boiling up fresh pasta or microwaving a bowl of porridge takes so little time I really wouldn't bother with shop-bought convenience foods. Save them for the weekend when you're off the diet.

5 basic foods

These five foods form the basis of my diet:
Potatoes, breakfast oats, fruit, fish and pasta

POTATOES

If I had to restrict my diet to one food, it would be potatoes. A much-maligned vegetable, potatoes have been eclipsed in recent years by the more trendy carbohydrate, pasta, but potatoes are powerhouses of nutrition which are cheap to buy, easy to grow and extremely versatile. A large potato only needs a scrub and it is ready to be cooked. It can be boiled, roasted, fried and baked. It can be filled, mashed and piped. Potatoes are excellent sources of starch, fibre, vitamin C, potassium and protein.

People think of potatoes as fattening, but they are not. It is the manner of cooking potatoes which raises the calorie content, but a potato on its own contains just twenty-five calories an ounce (30g). Freshly dug potatoes contain the most vitamin C, though boiling reduces the amount considerably. Mashed potatoes contain the least vitamin C. Frying actually preserves most of the vitamin, as does roasting.

People tend to think of chips as unhealthy junk food, when in fact they are highly nutritious, especially when fried in vegetable oils.

A WORD OF WARNING: Never eat green potatoes, or potatoes which are sprouting. They contain alkaloids such as solanine, which are highly poisonous even in small amounts and can cause migraine.

Oats are a wonderful source of soluble fibre, which has been linked to lower cholesterol levels. You will be eating a bowl of breakfast oats every morning and as a snack throughout the day, if desired. Most of the leading brands of oats contain the whole oat, which includes some bran, but in a bowl of cereal there is very little bran, so it will not cause the irritation that a serving of pure bran might trigger.

Oats are low in saturated fat, low in sodium, and if they are made with milk, they provide just under half your daily recommended intake of protein.

Their supply of complex carbohydrates are released over a period of about four hours, which means you feel satisfied and less hungry for longer than a sugary breakfast cereal.

FRUIT

BANANAS Bananas are one of nature's true convenience foods, which is why, apart from their nutritional value, they are included as a major ingredient of this diet. They come in their own packaging which keeps them hygienic and easy to pop into a pocket or bag. They contain potassium which is lost through perspiration and are thus invaluable for sports people or regular exercisers. They contain fibre, starch and natural sugars which are released into the bloodstream quickly, and which give an instant energy lift. I also use bananas as an easy base for milkshakes and desserts.

APPLES, GRAPES, BLACKCURRANTS, STRAWBERRIES, ETC. It goes without saying that any good diet includes fresh fruit. High in vitamin C, potassium and fibre, fruit also contains antioxidants which are linked to protection against cancer.

On this diet plan, apples and grapes will be eaten on their own or in a fruit salad, and we will also use rhubarb, blackcurrants, blackberries, gooseberries, etc. as purées, depending on the season.

A good winter fruit salad includes dried apricots, blackberries and prunes.

STRAWBERRIES High in vitamin C, with amounts of potassium and vitamins B1, B2 and B6, strawberry seeds contain lignin, a dietary fibre which is particularly effective at maintaining your digestive system. On this diet, only eat strawberries after 6pm, due to the laxative effect of the insoluble fibre.

FISH

Salmon, tuna fish and white fish such as cod are all high on my list of diet foods. Tinned tuna requires no preparation whatever and is ideal for either plain salads, sandwich fillings or for eating with jacket potatoes. Fresh salmon is something I like because it can be all things to all people! You can poach it and have it cold with a little mayonnaise, you can use it in sandwiches, or you can add a luscious hollandaise sauce, a few new potatoes and some asparagus and call it a formal dinner.

Tuna and salmon are high in Omega-3 fatty acids (which are essential as the body is unable to manufacture them), and though the general fat content is several times higher than for white fish, it is good fat, so you should not worry. The protein content is high and the calories low, at around fifty-five calories per ounce (30g) for salmon fillet and twenty-eight to fifty-four calories for tuna.

SMOKED SALMON Smoked salmon is particularly handy on diets because all you have to do is unwrap it, arrange it on a plate and top it with a squeeze of lemon and some freshly ground black pepper. Butter a slice of brown bread and *voilà!* – you have an easy light lunch or snack with only about 220 calories.

Smoked salmon has only 142 calories per $3^1/_2$oz/100g, is full of protein, iron and vitamin D, and has just 4.5g of essential fats.

PRAWNS Shellfish are a dieter's dream food. Low in fat and high in protein, they are rich in the B vitamins, selenium and iodine.

A WORD OF WARNING: Shellfish can trigger allergic reactions in some people, and as they are cooked in salted water they can be high in sodium and therefore should be avoided or kept to a minimum consumption by people who suffer from high blood pressure.

SARDINES Sardines are the only food which has more calcium than milk, as we eat the bones and skin too. One portion of sardines contains your entire day's intake of calcium, plus good amounts of protein, iron and zinc. Choose sardines which are canned in tomato sauce and enjoy an old favourite, sardines on toast.

PASTA

Pasta is not a high-calorie food. It can be used as the base for a great variety of dishes, and it is the topping or sauce which can contain the higher number of calories and turn a pasta dish into a fattening meal.

Made from wheat flour and water, the complex carbohydrates pasta provides are broken down by the body and used to build up stores of glycogen, or energy.

Pasta is also a source of protein, and it is low in fat. Some pastas are enriched with eggs, or have a range of additions which make them colourful, such as tomatoes and spinach.

Pasta is eaten every day on this diet. It is not only nutritious and filling, but it will keep your stomach flat because its starch content is very settling and uncontroversial for your digestion.

In addition, you will be eating a selection of the following:

AVOCADO PEARS I never understand why people are so fearful of avocados. They are the most delicious fruit, easy on the stomach and versatile. Half an avocado pear contains between 130 and 160 calories, depending on size, and it has the highest protein content of any fruit. It is high in potassium and vitamins C and E. Avocados also contain antioxidants which guard against damage by free radicals.

BEEF, LEAN Despite recent concern over the health of our beef cattle, this meat contains most of the nutrients needed by our bodies, with the exception of fibre. It contains protein, iron and zinc, and even vitamin C and calcium. Lean beef contains only fifty-five calories per ounce (30g).

BRAN CEREAL Bran itself has no nutritional value and it passes through our gut without being absorbed. However, for general health and to ward off the cancers associated with the stomach and to guard against diverticulitis and constipation, you should eat some high-fibre cereals. Always take with extra fluids.

BREAD Bread has been rising in popularity in recent years. Once seen as a stodgy staple food which came in either dry brown or unhealthy white, most supermarkets now carry a stunning array of bread which in addition to the better-known wholemeal and granary varieties now include continental types such as naan, pitta, rye breads, tortillas and focaccia – to name but a few. The addition of sun-dried tomatoes, olives and so forth to what are otherwise plain tin loaves has also raised the stock of bread to the slightly more trendy, all of which is to the good of our health.

If you can get it, I recommend a good white loaf made with unbleached flour, and it's worth hunting around for. Local small bakers often make it, and although it can be more expensive than conventional factory loaves, bread is still a cheap staple food and a slice of bread costs pennies.

Bread is a good source of protein and starch, and it is therefore excellent for vegetarians who cannot get their protein from animal sources. It also contains the B vitamins, calcium and iron. White bread might not contain all the fibre of wholemeal, but it contains twice as much calcium. By law, breads must be fortified. Wholemeal bread has more iron than white bread, and granary bread has malt flour added, and kernels of wheat to give it that 'nutty' texture.

Calorie contents do not vary much between breads, being roughly sixty to seventy per ounce (30g).

CHICKEN Chicken is a highly versatile food, which can be used as a base for a variety of dishes from a plain roast to an Indian curry.

Chicken is an excellent source of protein, and it also contains the B vitamins, some iron and zinc. Despite its animal origin, chicken does not contain much saturated fat, as much of the fat is under the skin, which can be removed before cooking. On The Standard Diet I have kept to plain grilled or roast chicken dishes, but on The Maintenance Plan it is extended to include the more exotic and spicy recipes.

DRIED FRUIT I have used dried fruit such as sultanas and raisins sparingly in this diet, mostly as a topping for evening suppers of cereal or yoghurt, but I have kept their quantities small due to their high sugar content. Remember, dried fruits are NOT fattening any more than any other food is fattening – it is the amount you eat which is the vital factor in weight control. However, because dried fruit adds sweetness without using refined sugar, and because of its high fibre and potassium content, it should be included in your daily diet.

EGGS The whole cholesterol question has become confusing for most people because it is linked to heart disease. Cholesterol is absolutely essential for the body for a variety of reasons which already fill several medical textbooks and which are beyond the scope of this book. However, two sources of cholesterol are cheese and eggs and taken in small quantities they will do you no harm at all. Eggs are cheap and easy to cook, and can form the basis of a huge range of meals. The white of an egg is pure protein with no fat at all, so the sugar apart, a meringue is one sweet item which will do you no harm. Bodybuilders eat a massive number of egg whites for their pure protein and muscle-building properties.

LIVE YOGHURT Live yoghurt is wonderful at calming the gut when you are suffering from bacterial activity which is causing wind and flatulence. I have used yoghurt for many of the desserts over the five days of the diet, and you should find that with the addition of either stewed fruit, or dried fruits and nuts, you will soon get used to the taste of this creamy, natural yoghurt. Yoghurt is a source of calcium and the B vitamins.

MILK Milk is versatile, cheap and highly necessary in any good diet. Women should drink plenty of milk for the health of their bones, and it has long been regarded as an essential for beauty. I use skimmed milk because I prefer the less creamy taste and find it refreshing, but by all means use semi-skimmed if you prefer. Milk is high in calcium, protein and vitamins and is known as nature's 'complete food'.

NUTS The same rules apply for nuts. Why people become hysterical at the thought of a handful of peanuts I will never understand, because they contain protein and many other nutrients. Yes, they contain a lot of calories per ounce which is why I only use a few, but do not cut out nuts from your diet completely. They are extremely good for you.

RICE Rice is a gluten-free carbohydrate, so it is suitable for people with coeliac disease. The starch in rice is digested and absorbed slowly, thus providing a steady release of glucose into the bloodstream. Eating rice has long been thought to be good for digestive disorders. On this diet you will eat rice both as a savoury and in the sweet pudding form.

VEGETABLES, DARK GREEN, SUCH AS BEANS, LETTUCE AND WATERCRESS These are the only green vegetables that are included on this diet, but they are more than enough for five days. Lambs' lettuce and watercress are used as a garnish for your lunches and sandwiches; French beans will be eaten with your evening meals.

All vegetables which are green and leafy contain valuable vitamin K which is essential for blood clotting and the formation of some proteins. They also contain folic acid, vitamin C and iron.

VEGETABLES, SALAD You will see that I usually describe salads as colourful. If you are having a warm salad for your meal you might be better off with a mixed green salad, but a colourful mix of salad vegetables gives you a wider range of nutrients, including betacarotene. This is what gives vegetables their colour, and betacarotene supplies us with vitamin A, which you would not get from green leaves alone. When you make your colourful salad, use sweetcorn, red, green and yellow peppers and grated carrots.

These are the foods that you will be eating over the next five days, and I hope you find plenty in there which is to your liking! I have sworn by these foods for many years whenever a flat stomach and high energy are vital, and have kept my fancy and exotic fruit diets for holiday times when I am relaxing.

Do bear one thing in mind. We would all prefer to eat exactly what we like and not to have to pick off skin, drain fat or weigh things. Unfortunately very few people can get away with that kind of regime and still look wonderful. If they don't suffer a weight problem they probably have a bad skin, weak nails or dry hair. If they look wonderful on a rubbishy diet and are in their twenties, rest assured it will catch up with them in their thirties or forties.

Nobody has less time for food fads than me. I detest pretentiousness about food and dieting, and I never believe anyone who says she prefers a slice of low-fat spinach roulade to a whopping wedge of double-choc-chip, double-cream Black Forest gâteau. The secret is to have your goal in your sights and learn not to mind. Looking good doesn't come easily, but it's worth the effort. Dieting may not be fun, but the results are. Keep that in your mind, and remember that the discipline is ALWAYS worth it.

A quick guide to nutrition

A common misconception is that if you want to eat healthy, nutritious food, you have to spend money on fancy gourmet foods. In fact, as long as you satisfy your body's needs for the right balance of carbohydrates, proteins and fats, you needn't spend more than a few pounds a week, a lot less than you would if you consistently snacked on chocolate and take-aways.

This diet is particularly satisfying because it contains a high proportion of bulky foods, such as potatoes, bread and pasta, which keep hunger pangs at bay for hours. It is vital for any dieter to eat plenty of carbohydrate.

CARBOHYDRATES

Carbohydrates fall into two categories, simple and complex. I've already told you about simple carbohydrates which are sugars, and complex carbohydrates, which are both fibre and starch. On this diet you will be eating a lot of starch, so it's as well to understand it:

STARCH

Starch is the major source of energy in this diet. Starchy foods contain no more calories per ounce than lean meat, and they should be the staple foods in all diets. Everything else is based on them.

Starchy foods
Bread, potatoes, rice, pasta, cereals

On this diet we will have portions of at least four out of the five starches in this list, every day. Later in the book you will see that I have classified most of the main meals into beef recipes or chicken recipes and so on. Your potato, rice and pasta dishes are similarly classified, and I think you will find such a tasty range of choices, which are very simple to shop for and prepare, that you will stick to them over a much longer period than that covered by this diet plan.

THE IMPORTANCE OF VARIETY

It is important that any diet is varied, both from the point of view of nutritional balance and to keep boredom at bay. So, while potatoes are undoubtedly good for you, and a staple of this diet, you wouldn't want to eat them three times a day. Similarly, you would get fed up of twelve slices of bread a day or sixteen oranges! The day-by-day eating plans come later in the book, but a suggested balance of foods would be something like this:

Breakfast One serving oats
Mid-morning One slice bread
Lunch One serving pasta or rice
Evening meal One or two servings potatoes, vegetables and fruit
Supper High-fibre cereal

If you have coeliac disease (gluten intolerance)

Potatoes and rice are wheat-free, and your cereals can be either corn flakes or Rice Crispies.

5 DAYS TO A FLATTER STOMACH

Every cell in the human body needs protein. Without it, tissue cannot be repaired effectively, nor can new cells grow. If you starve yourself on diets which give you hardly anything to eat, you are also doing a disservice to your looks and beauty. Proteins such as keratin and collagen keep your skin supple and young-looking, and your hair strong and elastic. Protein also helps fight infection and aids digestion.

You will be nourished by a good balance of protein on this diet, although only about 20 per cent of our daily nutritional requirements come from protein.

PROTEINS COME FROM TWO SOURCES – PLANTS AND ANIMALS

These are found in all foods from an animal source, such as:-

ANIMAL PROTEINS		PLANT PROTEINS	
Cheese	Fish	Wheat	Beans
Meat	Poultry	Bread	Potatoes
Milk	Eggs	Rice	Nuts

A drawback to proteins is that they cannot be stored by the body and are therefore taken to the liver and converted to glucose. If your diet is too rich in protein – for example if you are a big cheese or meat eater – you run the risk of osteoporosis because strange as it may seem, when you are eating calcium from cheese, too much protein can result in *loss* of calcium.

On your 5-day plan you will be eating most of the proteins listed above, with the exception of beans, and with only a very small amount of nuts, which you do not need to eat in quantity anyway. Just two Brazil nuts every day provides the average body with all it needs of some minerals such as selenium, and it also provides useful amounts of fat. A simple bowl of cereal with milk provides roughly a third of our daily recommended protein intake, so it is unlikely these days that many of us are deficient in protein.

FATS

Fat is essential in any good diet. Without it, vitamins A, D and E cannot be absorbed from the gut, and you can become severely vitamin deficient, leading to illness. Fats form every membrane in every cell of the human body. It is vital that you do not exclude fat from your everyday meals.

Like proteins, fats also come from two sources – plant and animal. The 'fat question' will always be a burning issue and hot topic of conversation, and ignorance is usually the cause, so here is a breakdown of the types of fat in our foods:

ANIMAL FATS
The so-called bad fats, found in:
Cheese, eggs, milk, meat

In fact, all these foods were in our list of proteins. The saturated fat contained in these foods is considered to be bad for the health of your heart. A rule of thumb is that if the fat is the type that solidifies when cooled after heating, it is less good for you. Unsaturated fat, like olive oil, sunflower oil and oil from nuts is generally thought to be better for health, although it does not make any difference when considering the question of weight loss, as all fats contain the same number of calories per ounce.

VEGETABLE FATS
Vegetable fats are mainly oils which contain a high proportion of unsaturated fatty acids.

SATURATED AND UNSATURATED
Fats are made up of fatty acids. There are two main types of fats, saturated and unsaturated. The unsaturated fats are then divided into *mono*unsaturated and *poly*unsaturated. Saturated fats are solid at room temperature – such as butter – and are found in most animal sources, such as eggs, milk and meat. Unsaturated fats are liquid, such as sunflower oil. Both saturated and monounsaturated fatty acids can be manufactured by the body from carbohydrates, alcohol and protein, so it is not essential to take extra supplies. Sources of saturated and monounsaturated fats include avocados, nuts, seeds, olive oil and fish oils.

Some polyunsaturated fatty acids cannot be made by the body and must therefore be taken in the form of the foods which contain them. These fatty acids are therefore called 'essential', and are made up of two groups called Omega-6 (found in vegetable oils) and Omega-3 (found in soya bean oil, rapeseed oil, sardines, herrings, mackerel and salmon).

An adult requires about 4g of Omega-6 fatty acids a day (a handful of almonds or two teaspoons of sunflower oil) with a maximum of 25g. Very high intakes may be harmful. Omega-3 fatty acids are needed in small amounts, 1–2g a day (a handful of walnuts or a small portion of oily fish). Deficiency in either fatty acid can lead to poor growth, skin problems and a weakened immune system.

It is important to understand that all fats can cause you to gain weight. When eaten in excess, even the so-called 'good' fats, the essential fatty acids found in fish and vegetable oils, will cause you to gain weight. If your total intake of calories – from whatever source – exceeds the number you use in energy expenditure every day, *the excess will be stored as fat*.

Certain vitamins can only be absorbed with the assistance of fat, so a fat-free diet is extremely disadvantageous to your health. Healthy adults need about 30g of fat a day in order that the body can absorb vitamins A, D and E.

TRANSFATS

Transfats are added to products to prevent them becoming hard and rancid. Look out for 'hydrogenated' on labels, such as margarine. Mainly found in processed foods such as crisps, cakes and biscuits.

On this diet you will not need to concern yourself with transfats as I avoid processed foods and stick with fresh. The milk in this diet will be skimmed or semi-skimmed and unless you are a vegetarian you will be eating lean beef and poultry. On the whole, you should not avoid fats, but try not to use them unnecessarily, such as spreading thick layers of butter on your bread or by piling it into your jacket potato! Popular belief is that removing all the fat from a diet will prevent the formation of body fat. If only that were true, we'd all be doing it, we'd all be slim and the diet industry would vanish overnight! Cutting out fat will not stop you gaining body fat, and I'm afraid that the simple answer is that if you eat more calories of food than your body needs – whether in salads, oats, chocolate or apples – you will put on weight. Simple!

There is no doubt that saturated fat is bad for you in quantity. However, try not to get hysterical and cut out the things you enjoy in life, and do remember that foods such as cheese and eggs are extremely good for your looks. A cheese and pickle sandwich or a boiled egg and soldiers are surely two of life's simple pleasures, and denying yourself the things you like is faddy and hysterical. If cheese made you fat, everyone who eats it would be fat. If banning it guaranteed weight loss, why are so many people who eat low-fat diets still overweight?

Fat is a necessary part of any good diet, but the key to healthy eating and weight loss is the *percentage* of your daily diet which fats make up. Experts disagree but a sensible level would be no more than 20 per cent of your diet. This is easy to calculate if you keep a food diary for a week.

Vitamins and minerals

Each individual will have different nutritional needs, but it is fair to say that guidelines can be set for the average man or woman who is in good health, regardless of occupation, age or size. The only adjustments which need to be taken into account are for extreme juvenile or senile individuals, for pregnant or nursing mothers or for those engaged in particularly strenuous physical activity, such as professional sportspeople, dancers or manual workers.

Vitamins are usually classed as water- or fat-soluble. Water-soluble vitamins are all the B vitamins and vitamin C, and they cannot be stored by the body as any excess is excreted in the urine. Thus, a person who takes a massive amount of vitamin C each day in the hope that it will be stored to ward off a cold is wasting money. Never take too many vitamins as they can be poisonous to the system. Always read the label on the bottle.

Vitamins A, D, E and K are fat-soluble, which means

that they need an intake of fat to be effective. Unlike water-soluble vitamins these are stored by the body which means that any excess can be highly dangerous for your health. There is a list of vitamins and their food sources and how much your body needs each day on pages 92–93.

ESSENTIAL MINERALS

A balanced diet will also include adequate amounts of calcium and iron among other trace elements and minerals, and it is important to know their sources.

Vegetarians and vegans, in particular, have need of non-meat sources of iron, vitamin B12 and folates.

IRON Sources include pulses, oatmeal, wholemeal bread, nuts, parsley, egg yolks and fortified breakfast cereals
CALCIUM Milk and butter, cheese, nuts, sunflower seeds, soya products and leafy vegetables
FOLATE Leafy vegetables, beans, eggs, peanuts, fruit, wholegrain cereals

Iron is lost through perspiration, so supplements might be needed if you exercise a lot. Other minerals such as iodine and manganese, known as trace elements, are needed in tiny amounts, while potassium, sodium, calcium and magnesium are needed in quite large quantities. However, on this diet, you will be eating all you require of these minerals.

Fat is a neccesary part of any good diet, but the key to healthy eating and weight loss is the *percentage* of your daily which fats make up. Experts disagree but a sensible level would be no more than 20 per cent of your diet. This is easy to calculate if you keep a food diary for a week.

VITAMIN SUPPLEMENTS

Should you be taking extra vitamins or mineral supplements on this diet? Many people pop dozens of pills every day without the slightest idea of what they are taking or whether they need them, and you may not know that some vitamins are highly toxic taken in large doses on a regular basis. Others, such as vitamin C, can't be stored by the body, so excess is simply excreted through the urine, which is literally money

VITAMIN	SOURCES	DAILY REQUIREMENT
Vitamin A Comes from retinol found in animal foods or betacarotene, found in plant foods	Carrots, red/yellow/ green peppers, egg yolks, liver, butter, cheese, oily fish	700mcg for men 600mcg for women (Equivalent to about 2oz/50g carrots or one small slice of liver)
Vitamin B1	Potatoes, liver, kidneys, cereals, nuts, beans, peas	1mg for men 0.8mg for women (Approx 4 tbsp rice or seven pieces wholemeal bread per day)
Vitamin B2 (riboflavin)	Poultry, fish, milk, eggs, meat, some cereals	1.3mg for men 1.1mg for women (One bowl cereal provides half daily requirement)
Vitamin B6 (pyridoxine)	Nuts, bananas, yeast, poultry, fish, fortified breakfast cereals, eggs, soya beans	1.4mg for men 1.2mg for women (One serving fish or two bowls cereal will provide an adequate daily intake)
Vitamin B12	Meat, poultry, eggs, fish, dairy products	1.5mcg for men 1.5mcg for women (Enough B12 will be derived from one glass of milk or a serving of meat or fish)
Niacin (nicotinic acid)	Pulse vegetables, lean meat, poultry, potatoes, nuts, cereals	17mg for men 13mg for women (Derived from protein, one serving of meat, poultry or fish will provide the recommended daily intake)

VITAMIN	SOURCES	DAILY REQUIREMENT
Folate (folic acid)	Liver, dark green leafy vegetables, bread, cereals, cruciferous vegetables	200mcg for men and women (Two servings vegetables provide daily requirement, or four glasses fresh orange juice)
Vitamin C	Fruits and vegetables including peppers and potatoes	40mcg for men and women (One apple, orange, peach or potato)
Vitamin D	Sardines, tuna fish, eggs, salmon, cereals	About 10mcg, although the body manufactures vitamin D from sunlight, so deficiency is rare (One serving of sardines or tuna fish provides the recommended daily intake)
Vitamin E	Wheatgerm, vegetable oils, margarines, nuts, seeds, fish oils	3–4mg for men and women (A handful of nuts would supply enough for a good daily intake)
Vitamin K	Dark green leafy vegetables	70mcg for men 65mcg for women (One serving of leafy vegetables a day)

down the drain. It makes sense to question whether we really need extra vitamins, or whether our diet is sufficient in itself to satisfy our daily requirements.

It goes without saying that your food intake should contain all that you need in the way of nutrients. What most people don't realize, however, is that these nutrients are lost in different ways and at different rates according to our lifestyles, and no two people's needs are the same.

Take a sedentary, young and single office worker who lives at home and has all the household worries shouldered by her parents. Stress and anxiety count for the loss of many nutrients from the body, as does an active lifestyle, so this type of person could have less need of extra vitamins and minerals. But what if she smokes? Did you know that you lost 25mg (¾oz) of vitamin C *every time* you light up? Cigarette smoking inhibits the absorption of vitamin C, as does the polluted atmosphere of an inner city, so if this is you, you'll need a supplement.

Coffee and tea drinking also inhibit absorption of vitamins, so if you drink a lot of these, either cut down, change to the caffeine-free varieties or take extra vitamins. The small amount of vitamins you are losing may not seem much, but remember that the effect is cumulative. If you drink caffeine a little, have the odd cigarette, drink alcohol daily, live in the city and have a pressured life, you are already beginning to store up trouble. If you add to this a diet of junk food, missed meals and lack of sleep, you need to seriously consider your long-term health. The point is, we can all get away with it while we are young. We can smoke, drink and party all night, and still bounce out of bed in the morning looking fabulous. Wait a few years, though, and you'll have a different tale to tell, and I know many dozens of women who speak of their past excesses with regret. You don't want to live like a hermit on bread and water, but neither do you want to end up in a few years' time with a bad back and aching joints, simply because you took no exercise and ate rubbish.

It goes without saying that an active lifestyle, such as a factory or agricultural worker means that the demands on your body are greater than for the sedentary worker. Keen exercisers, too, need extra iron as much of it is lost through sweating, and of course strict slimmers should take a multi-vitamin and mineral supplement every day.

If you drink alcohol heavily, not only are you damaging your health through dehydration and liver toxicity, but you could be in danger of a deficiency of thiamine (vitamin B1) which is needed to convert carbohydrates and fats into energy. Symptoms include lethargy, muscle weakness and numbness.

As I have said, vitamin A can be toxic and extremely hazardous to health in quantity. Pregnant women should avoid eating liver for this reason, and should never take a vitamin A supplement due to possible damage to the unborn baby.

If you have been used to what might be called an unhealthy or junk-food diet, this 5-day plan will be a breath of fresh air to your system with its supplies of fresh foods, plenty of starch for energy, fibre, protein and essential fats, plus of course the all-important water content which your body will thank you for. Because we all have different needs due to age and lifestyle, I suggest you go and buy just one bottle of multivitamins with minerals, and take one a day. You will come to no harm, and any excess will simply be excreted.

If you find it hard to be bothered to take extra vitamins for the sake of your health, do it for your looks. A sallow skin, dull hair and brittle nails are unattractive, yet they can be easily dealt with by eating a good diet which supplies all the correct nutrients. Don't get hung up about it, but do bear it in mind.

Portion control

At the very beginning of this book I said that it wasn't the food which made you fat, it was how much of it you ate. No food is fattening, and you must never approach any slimming diet with the attitude 'what can I eat a lot of?' Why not? Because while there is nothing wrong with a genuine love of food, and I wholly endorse the attention we should pay to special meals, the psychological distress caused by being fat and feeling unattractive far outweighs the benefits of those few moments of pleasure when we eat more than we really want.

A specific psychological factor in our eating patterns is the being good factor. 'I've been good, I only had one portion of ice-cream' said a friend the other day. 'I was really naughty last night' said another, 'I had a whole bottle of wine and *two* puddings – then I tucked into all the chocolate mints!' Now why do we call eating less 'good' and eating more 'bad'? And why do we genuinely feel better because we managed to say no to a second helping?

If you are to have a flatter stomach, you must eat smaller portions and tell yourself that you can eat whatever treat you think you may be missing at any time you like. People eat too much to make the most of the opportunity. As you will have seen, one vital factor in the size of your stomach is the size and regularity of your meals. It is no good having a couple of substantial meals a day and nothing in between. Eat little and often.

I have three pieces of kitchen equipment which have been invaluable to me over the years. The first is my blender, with which I can make all the mousses and milkshakes which are so much a part of this diet, and the second is a set of food weighing scales which I bought over twenty years ago. They are large scales – in other words they weigh by the quarter ounce (8g) and only go up to eight ounces (225g). On conventional scales it is easy to add half an ounce without knowing it, but these scales are incredibly accurate. You don't need to be obsessed with weighing everything, but if you are very overweight you will find them invaluable. I also find that their accuracy guarantees the success of temperamental recipes. Finally, I use an igloo scoop for my purée and mashed vegetable servings – the sort which were used to serve up mashed potatoes at school years ago – and quite apart from the fact that they make carrots and puréed greens look rather ritzy, you know how much you are getting. I do recommend that you buy a scoop to help your portion control.

Three basic important rules are to eat every three hours, not to skip breakfast or a snack at bedtime and to drink water plentifully.

BREAKFAST

Your breakfast every day will be either porridge or two slices of toast with a little butter from your ration. Use ordinary breakfast oats or the jumbo oats if you prefer a coarser consistency to the stodgier feel of the normal, smaller oats. It's purely a matter of taste.

Simply take 1oz/30g of oats, place in either a pan or a microwave dish and cover with water. Again, the consistency is a matter of personal preference and you will have to experiment a little, so adjust the water to suit yourself.

Microwave for two and a half minutes or simmer in a pan for two minutes once boiled. Add a little skimmed milk if you like, though I prefer it without. Allow to cool, and add either a teaspoonful of sugar or half a teaspoon of golden syrup.

If you are having toast, use unbleached white bread from a good baker.

VEGETABLES

Healthy though they are, do not fall into the trap of allowing yourself unlimited vegetables. Vegetable portions are always just two tablespoonfuls or a scoop of mashed vegetables. If you are having potatoes as an accompanying vegetable, use just one medium-sized potato (4oz/125g), or two small new potatoes, or a scoop of mashed.

SALADS

Never have a massive salad just to fill up. It encourages gluttony. A salad is four or five leaves of lettuce, one chopped tomato, three or four slices of cucumber, a spoonful of sweetcorn, a spoonful of grated carrot and one slice each of red, green and yellow peppers. A sprig or two of watercress finishes the salad.

CHICKEN DISHES

Use one chicken breast for your chicken meals. I have given most of the meal suggestions for one portion only, except where it would be impractical to make a particular dish for one portion only, so double or treble the quantities if you wish to share your meals or have three or more to cater for.

PASTA OR RICE

All pasta and rice meals are 2oz/60g dry weight using fresh pasta. It doesn't seem much, but you will get used to it. If you are very hungry and decide to have more, try eating the amount I have suggested and keeping the extra portion hot as a second helping. Wait ten minutes after you have finished and ask yourself if you really still want it.

BREAD

One medium slice from a ready-sliced loaf.

RICE PUDDING AND OTHER PUDDINGS

A guide to your desserts and puddings is that the amount you have should fit into a standard yoghurt pot (5oz/150g).

STEWED FRUITS

Stew apples, gooseberries, plums and blackberries etc. with a small amount of sugar to taste, if you simply cannot bear it unsweetened. I can't. On no account use artificial sweeteners. A teaspoon of sugar is negligible in calorie terms, and tastes much nicer than the chemical alternatives.

FISH

Use a standard sized fillet of salmon, cod or your chosen fish (about 4–6oz/125–180g in weight). Always poach or grill the fish, except for the one recipe for fried salmon where butter is used. Much of the butter is left at the bottom of the pan, and knowing you are having it will encourage you to go easy.

BUTTER TOPPINGS

Butter is used sparingly on this diet, but do not use low-fat alternatives as they are really not worth the calorie savings and contain a lot of undesirable additives. The ration for five days is 2oz/60g and I suggest you weigh it out and keep it in a separate little dish.

MILK

As you will be drinking skimmed milk, use as much as you like in tea or coffee, and I have suggested 45fl oz/100ml for your milkshakes and evening cereal snacks. If you really can't stand the idea of skimmed milk, use semi-skimmed.

3

Standard 5-Day Plan

....

This plan should be followed for 5 days only. For the two days following you can either stick to it by returning to day one, or relax a little while still keeping with the general principles. No doubt you will have times when your eating is erratic, such as at the weekend or if you are staying away from home, but by remembering your portion control, your three-hour limit and the rule about drinking water with every meal, I believe you will manage to avoid temptation better than you may have done in the past.

ADVANCE PREPARATION

Everybody is busy, so anything which you can prepare in advance helps you stay away from temptation in the kitchen. Here are some suggestions:

1. It's a good idea to make a rice pudding in advance (see p.151). You can pot it up into empty yoghurt cartons and take one to work.

2. Where possible, I have suggested you make two of something and keep one portion for the next day. An example is the poached salmon (p.133) and grilled chicken breast (p.128), which are both nice to have cold in sandwiches or salads, and are so time-saving for working people or busy parents.

3. Always have a hard-boiled egg and grated cheese handy in the fridge.

4. Weigh out your ration of butter and put it in a separate dish in the fridge ready for use. This is 2oz/60g for five days (or 3oz/90g for a week).

WHAT IF I DON'T LIKE SOMETHING?

Some foods, such as bananas, are suggested quite frequently for snacks, and I agree that if you don't like them you can seem to be stuck. The fact is, any high-starch snack will do just as well, and I'd rather you had a piece of bread, toast or even cold potatoes than give in and eat sweets or chocolate. Don't snack on apples, citrus fruit or raw vegetables, especially if you have a problem with bloating. Stick to high-starch, filling foods, with plenty of water to sip.

The whole point is that as time goes by you'll get the hang of the principles of this diet plan and will be able to adapt it to suit yourself. I know you'll find the high-starch plan works, and you'll soon be able to add or subtract meals which are your personal favourites. For the time being though, stick directly with the first five days – then go on to adapt The Maintenance Plan.

DAY 1

BREAKFAST
one portion porridge, made with 1oz/30g of oats and water
a teaspoon of golden syrup, if desired
OR
one or two slices of toast with butter from the allowance

one glass mineral water
tea or coffee, as preferred

MID-MORNING
glass of banana milkshake
(one medium banana blended with 4fl oz/100ml skimmed
milk – this can be made at home and taken to work)
OR
one toasted crumpet, butter from the allowance

water

MID-DAY MEAL
PASTA WITH LEMON AND DILL (p.139 – this can be
cooked in advance and taken to work as a cold salad, either
on its own or with 1oz/30g of tuna fish)
OR
tuna fish with mashed potatoes
(half a tin of drained tuna fish with 6oz/180g potatoes,
boiled and mashed with skimmed milk, salt and pepper)

MID-AFTERNOON
one pot of live bio-yoghurt

EVENING MEAL

POACHED OR GRILLED FILLET OF SALMON OR COD
(p.133)
OR
VEGETABLE PAELLA (P.141)
mixed fruit salad with half an apple, half a banana, six
grapes, six strawberries, sliced apricots, raspberries, etc.

SUPPER (OPTIONAL)
one Weetabix or Shredded Wheat
4fl oz/100ml skimmed milk
two Brazil nuts, flaked, or a few flaked almonds (optional)

glass of water
tea or decaffeinated coffee
bedtime drink

YOUR EXERCISES TODAY

1. Start the day with your warm-up (p.46), mobilizing (p.51)
and stretch routine (p.52).
2. Go for a brisk walk if possible.
3. Do three minutes of abdominal exercises. Stick with The
Foundation exercise (p.58), which you should do for one set
of eight counts (one count being up and down), turn over
to stretch out, then repeat the process twice.
4. Lunchtime. Take a break and do twenty minutes of brisk
exercise. If you are at home, try ten minutes of dancing or
jogging on the spot to music, followed by the same set of
stomach exercises you did this morning.
5. Early evening. Try to go swimming or for a cycle ride if
the weather is fine. If you are doing this, save your larger
meal until afterwards, have your Weetabix or Shredded
Wheat now.
    Do your three minutes of stomach exercises.
6. Before bed. Do a simple stretch routine and three minutes
of stomach exercises. Finish with a good stretch to relax you
before sleeping.

DAY 2

BREAKFAST
porridge made with 1oz/30g of oats and water
OR
toast with butter from your allowance

glass of water
tea or coffee

MID-MORNING BREAK
one pot of RICE PUDDING (p.151)
OR
one banana

glass of water
tea or decaffeinated coffee

MID-DAY BREAK
cold salmon mayonnaise and 6oz/180g jacket potato (use the
salmon from last night and a dot of MAYONNAISE, see p.157)
OR
cold vegetarian alternative
OR
poached salmon sandwiches
(use the salmon from last night, two slices white unbleached
bread, butter from allowance and a dot of MAYONNAISE, see
p.157)
OR
cheese on toast or cheese sandwich
1oz/30g Edam cheese on one slice (toasted) bread
lightly buttered

glass of water
tea or coffee

MID-AFTERNOON BREAK
one slice bread and jam (1tsp jam)
OR
banana milkshake

EVENING MEAL
roast or grilled chicken breast
4oz/125g boiled potatoes
carrots
French beans or peas
2 tbsp Bisto gravy
(I suggest you cook two pieces of chicken and leave one
cold, for tomorrow)
OR
MUSHROOM STROGANOFF (p.144)
green salad
OR
(lighter meal)
WALDORF SALAD (p.146)

BANANA AND STRAWBERRY MOUSSE (p.153)
OR
WINTER FRUIT SALAD with 1tsp *crème fraîche* (see p.154)

SUPPER (OPTIONAL)
one slice wholemeal toast, butter from the allowance
one apple
bedtime drink

YOUR EXERCISES TODAY

1. As yesterday, start the morning with a good stretch (p.52) and go through your warm-up routine (p.46).
2. Do just three minutes of abdominal exercises, repeating The Foundation exercise (p.58) for two sets. Progress to two sets of The Waist Whittler (p.62), stretch out and repeat.
3. In the evening, try to get at least a twenty-minute brisk walk in, even if you only go round the block or take the dog out. If you feel lethargic during the evening, you'll sleep so much better if you make yourself go out, even if it's freezing outside. The fresh air will do you good.

I always do this when staying away from home, and even boring suburban areas can take on a new meaning when you put on your coat and stride out round the roads. Just get yourself moving, and the faster the better!

4. If, on the other hand, you have a proper sports centre nearby, make yourself go for a few lengths of the pool or a game of squash or tennis, if you can find a partner. I know that having to pack all that kit is a bore, but it's better than not doing anything.
5. If you are tied to the house, find somewhere quiet and spend just ten minutes on your warm-up, stretch and stomach exercises. Repeat as for this morning.

DAY 3

BREAKFAST
porridge
OR
one slice of toast, with butter from your allowance

glass of water
tea or coffee

MID-MORNING BREAK
one chicken, tuna fish or tomato sandwich
OR
one toasted plain muffin, butter from allowance

cup of tea or coffee
glass of water

MID-DAY BREAK
one fillet of smoked mackerel with bread and butter
OR
COLD PASTA WITH LEMON AND DILL (p.139)

one pot of bio-yoghurt
glass of water
cup of tea or coffee

MID-AFTERNOON BREAK
one pot RICE PUDDING (p.152)
OR
banana milkshake

EVENING MEAL
HERB OMELETTE (p.142)
a colourful mixed salad of tomatoes, red and green peppers,
grated carrots, one sliced tomato, lettuce, watercress, rocket
and sweetcorn

OR
one portion of SHEPHERD'S PIE (p.125)
2 tbsp runner beans or peas
2 tbsp puréed carrots
stewed apple and blackberry
OR
fresh fruit salad

SUPPER (OPTIONAL)
1oz/30g bran flakes
4fl oz/100ml skimmed milk
bedtime drink

YOUR EXERCISES TODAY

1. You must practice your posture exercises today. However good you look, however slim you might be feeling, it's vital that you consider how you are standing and sitting to make the most of your flat stomach.
2. Try lying on the floor and stretching out your pectoral muscles (the chest muscles as described on page 68.)
3. Sit on a straight-backed chair and lean backwards. Let your mouth drop open. Take your arms behind the chair and clasp your hands. Pull backwards and downwards. Hold for ten seconds. Release and repeat.
4. Now to your stomach exercises. Try to do these three times today. Start with your Foundation Exercise (p.58). You should be able to do four sets by now. Rest and then repeat.
5. Turn over and stretch out.
6. Add in The Crunch (p.61) for four sets.
7. Stretch out.
8. Now do The Waist Whittler (p.62) for two sets each side.
9. Stretch out.
10. Add in two sets of The Chair Lift (p.64).
11. Stretch out. Well done.

How are you getting on with the diet? The most important thing to remember is that you are going to see results *very soon*, if you have not already. If you are craving one of your old fancies like a chocolate bar *don't give in!!* All your efforts over the past three days will be wasted.

5 DAYS TO A FLATTER STOMACH

DAY 4

BREAKFAST
porridge made with 1oz/30g of oats and water
OR
two slices of toast, with butter from your allowance

tea or coffee

MID-MORNING
one pot bio-yoghurt

MID-DAY BREAK
sardines on toast
OR
one 6oz/180g jacket potato
2 tbsp cottage cheese
OR
mixed salad sandwich – two slices unbleached white bread
with watercress, grated carrot, lettuce and cucumber

banana
glass of water
tea or coffee

MID-AFTERNOON BREAK
half an avocado pear eaten from the shell
tea or coffee

EVENING MEAL
PASTA PRIMAVERA (p.139)
OR
two grilled lamb chops, mint sauce
4oz/125g boiled potatoes
2 tbsp carrots, beans or peas
OR
WINTER SALAD (p.146)

SUPPER (OPTIONAL)

sliced fresh strawberries with milk and sugar

OR

stewed apple and blackberry with 1¹/₂ tbsp CUSTARD (p.158)

OR

apricot, prune and pear mix with 1¹/₂ tbsp CUSTARD (p.158)

handful of grapes
two Brazil nuts
glass of water
bedtime drink

YOUR EXERCISES TODAY

1. As always, start the day with your stretches and warm-up.

2. Today we're going to add The Air Bike (p.65).

a) Take position on the floor, for The Foundation exercise (p.58). Do two sets, pause and stretch and repeat the two sets again.

b) Progress to The Crunch (p.61). Do one or two sets (according to your fitness). Stretch and repeat.

c) Now add one set each side of The Waist Whittler (p.62). Stretch.

d) Move on to The Chair Lift (p.64). Do one or two sets of eight. Rest and repeat.

e) Now The Air Bike (p.65). Be careful as this is a difficult exercise, so definitely don't try it if you are new to exercise or very overweight. Don't despair though – you will get to it in time!

Do one set and rest, bringing your knees in to your chest. Now do two further sets. Stretch out.

3. Try to do some of these exercises in the middle of the day, and repeat the whole sequence before you have your evening meal.

4. Do your posture stretches before bed.

DAY
5

BREAKFAST
porridge made with 1oz/30g of oats and water
OR
one slice of toast
tea or coffee

MID-MORNING
one banana

MID-DAY BREAK
one 6oz/180g jacket potato
with 1oz/30g grated hard cheese and watercress
OR
one egg, poached, on one slice of toast
OR
half an avocado pear, sliced, mixed with either 3oz/90g
smoked chicken breast or one tomato and some raw grated
beetroot, and a few salad leaves, dressed with vinaigrette

MID-AFTERNOON BREAK
one pot live bio-yoghurt with one tsp stewed fruit
glass of water

EVENING MEAL
SPAGHETTI WITH SMOKED SALMON AND DILL (p.137)
colourful mixed salad with a little vinaigrette dressing
OR
grilled fillet of plaice
two boiled potatoes
2 tbsp carrots and runner/French beans
OR
(lighter meal)
COURGETTE, CARROT, GRAPEFRUIT AND AVOCADO SALAD
(p.147)
WINTER FRUIT SALAD (p.154)

OR
fresh fruit salad

SUPPER (OPTIONAL)
one slice wholemeal toast
coffee or tea
glass of water

YOUR EXERCISES TODAY

You have done really well so far on your diet plan, and if you've been following the exercises I've set you every day you should be feeling much more toned by now.

Today we're going to put all the exercises together for a slightly longer session, which will take about eight to ten minutes in total, depending on how fast the music is that you've chosen!

1. When you get up, do your usual warm-up and stretch.
2. Lie on the floor and get ready to do The Foundation exercise (p.58). Do two sets of eight, rest by bringing your knees into your chest, then repeat the two sets.
3. Turn over and stretch your spine.
4. Move on to The Crunch (p.61). Do two sets of eight, rest and repeat.
5. Stretch out.
6. Do one set each side of The Waist Whittler (p.62). Rest and Repeat.
7. Do one or two sets of The Chair Lift (p.64). Turn over and stretch your spine. Repeat the two sets.
8. Move on to The Air Bike (p.65). Remember, one count is left–right. Do two sets of eight. Rest and repeat.
9. Finally, if you can manage it, do one set of each exercise.
10. Turn over and give your spine a good stretch.

Well done! You have managed to get through five days of pretty hard exercise for your stomach muscles. Do keep it up. Have a day off tomorrow but go for a walk, go swimming or cycling, or simply get outside for a spot of gardening if you have a garden. Whatever you do, don't do nothing!

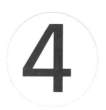

4

Where do I go from here?

....

You should be very pleased with your progress on the 5 Days to a Flatter Stomach plan. So where do you go from here? I have already suggested that for the next two days you simply relax the plan a little, but what does that mean? Well, rather than leave you to go mad for a couple of days, here are a few ideas which allow several of the missing foods from the 5-day plan. If any of them disagree with you however, go straight back to the starch-only regime.

Lunch can include a ploughman's lunch of bread, cheese and salad, but when ordering ask them to give you a bit less cheese and a bit more salad. You can also have thin and crispy-based pizza, a slice of quiche and salad or soups.

Evening meals out can be a bit more of a problem, but don't undo all your good work. Go for grilled steaks or chicken, potatoes and vegetables but be very careful about diving into the bread rolls and butter while you're waiting. Anything with fish as a starter or main course is always good, unless it is coated with batter or swimming in sauce. Don't ever be afraid to ask for something to be plain, or even to ask for a special dish. I was at a particularly ritzy hotel last year, and there was genuinely nothing on the menu I could stomach having just got over a tummy bug. 'You couldn't do me an omelette could you?' I implored, and they cheerfully did me the most wonderful omelette I've ever tasted.

Try this with puddings too. They've always got plenty of fruit in their kitchens and I usually ask if they've got a bit of fruit salad tucked away – they always have, or can do it for you. Otherwise if melon was on the menu as a starter, ask if you can have that. These places are there to make a living and would rather you went home telling your friends how obliging they were, so never feel backed into a corner by a fattening menu. Remember – plain food is far more chic and will help your looks far more than waistband-straining, spot-inducing fry-ups!

True to the principles of my diet, however, don't feel as if any foods are taboo. I have included the guidelines above because for many of us, one taste of a cake, chocolate or a few chips, and our diet is broken. If you feel you can control yourself, have anything you like but remember your portion control rules.

Drink wine, champagne or beer, but not liqueurs or aperitifs such as Campari, port or green Chartreuse, which are loaded with calories. Alcohol is all very well but it weakens your resolve, and before you know it you're shovelling in the food and undoing all your good work of last week. Stay off the peanuts too, because you'll never stick with just a handful!

If your Saturday night is going to be no more exciting than catching up with your ironing, don't worry. Use the time to steal a march on your girlfriends by sticking on a face mask and choosing one of the diet meals with a good glass of water – it's not *compulsory* to go out and drink everything in sight, and at least it won't be you who's agonizing over her spots and bloated stomach on Monday!

The Maintenance Plan

Remind yourself of the rules and guidelines on page 73.

IF YOU'RE A GUEST OR A HOSTESS

1. **Never** say you're on a diet, it just goads people into making a comment.

2. **Never** say 'only a little please' or 'just a small portion for me', it alerts people to the fact that you're being careful. Take whatever you're dished out, and play around with it, eating some and appearing to enjoy it.

3. **Never** worry about leaving food. You don't owe anybody an explanation of why you are not eating something, and if you are asked if the meal was all right, smile very brightly and say 'Yes thank you, it was delicious!'

4. **Don't** refuse anything unless you genuinely don't like it. Once everyone is into the swing of the evening they won't have a clue whether you've eaten it or not.

5. **If** you are the hostess, people will expect you to be busy, so I doubt that they will wonder if you are eating very little yourself. Don't comment on anybody else's eating habits – they could have a problem they'd rather not broadcast and could be embarrassed by close questioning, however well meant.

6. **Drink water** as you go. It will fill you up so you won't have any problem with refusing further helpings.

7. **Never** eat something simply because it's there. You aren't starving, and mustn't act as if you'll never get the chance to eat a certain dish ever again. Tell yourself that you can have it any time you want it, but not today. If you still want it tomorrow, tell yourself, you'll have it.

I promised you a diet of two speeds. I devised it because this is what people asked me for. If you just want to keep yourself in line, my Maintenance Plan is realistic about your wanting a few sweet things to eat, as too much denial only leads to cravings. You can have some alcohol too, though go easy as alcohol loosens your resolve to say no to food and yet more drink. An extra potato or slice of chicken isn't a problem, and I've suggested five cakes which have no fat in them and are relatively low-calorie. You can adapt the recipes for your own requirements.

KEEP UP THE GOOD WORK

You have only done five days of this diet, but you will have already found that not only does it work, that your stomach is feeling much, much flatter but that you need less food on your plate in order to feel satisfied. If you want to continue the diet for a further five days, go back to Day One, and either repeat the diet faithfully, or substitute a new evening meal or lunch each day from the five-meals recipe section. ALL the meals in this book are suitable for your diet; it is the size of PORTION that matters most in weight loss.

YOU **MUST** KEEP EXERCISING!

Your figure is important to you, and having a flat stomach feels wonderful. If you give up now, you'll be holding in your stomach for the rest of your life, choosing seats where your stomach is best hidden, wearing clothes you hate. You don't have to feel like that. But nobody can do it for you. For the sake of a little self-discipline and an extra walk every day, you can have the body of your dreams. *You can!*

No diet can exercise your muscles, so don't give up. If it is dark and cold and raining outside you might be tempted to stay in by the fire. DON'T! The fire is all the better to come back to if you have been out at a fitness class or having a game of badminton, or whatever. Remember, *losing weight is fine, but your figure matters too!* You don't want to get to summer and find that you're ashamed of your stomach because it's still flabby, despite having lost all that weight.

THE NEXT STEP

The next step is The Maintenance Diet, which I know you'll enjoy. I call this my 'free-range' diet because you have more choices. I hope you like it.

5 DAYS TO A FLATTER STOMACH

The Maintenance Diet

You are allowed two glasses of wine or champagne every day, or one glass of lager or beer. You should still drink plain mineral water with your meals and between them. Have a cake every day from the recipe list if you wish to, and you can start to introduce fruit during the day *as long as it doesn't bloat you!* Otherwise, stick to bananas.

DAY 1

BREAKFAST

one portion of porridge (make as before with 1oz/30g oats and water)

OR

one bowl Rice Crispies with 4fl oz/100ml skimmed milk
one egg, scrambled, on one slice toast
(try making the scrambled egg in a microwave oven)

MID-MORNING

one crumpet or bagel, toasted

OR

a sliced banana and apple, mixed

glass of water
tea or decaffeinated coffee

LUNCH

bowl of asparagus or vichyssoise soup and crusty bread
(I suggest you buy these soups; look out especially for the
New Covent Garden Soup Company brand)
OR
sliced avocado with either 4oz/125g prawns and
1tsp mayonnaise or 2 tbsp hummus with one slice of bread
and butter

one pot bio-yoghurt

MID-AFTERNOON

one round of toast and butter from allowance
OR
one cake from list (p.148)

EVENING MEAL

grilled fillet of plaice topped with pat of parsley butter and
lemon
OR
SPAGHETTI BOLOGNAISE (p.124)
OR
MUSHROOM STROGANOFF (p.144) with a green salad

APPLE OR RHUBARB SNOW (p.153)
OR
one portion RICE PUDDING (p.152)

SUPPER

1oz/30g bran flakes or Shredded Wheat
$^{1}/_{4}$ pint/150ml skimmed milk
handful of grapes
sliced strawberries
two flaked almonds or Brazil nuts
handful of wheatgerm

DAY 2

BREAKFAST
two slices of unbleached toast with butter and marmalade
tea or decaffeinated coffee
one 4fl oz/100ml glass fresh orange juice

MID-MORNING
banana and CUSTARD (p.158)

LUNCH
two rashers of back bacon, grilled, in a sandwich
OR
tuna and pasta salad
(2oz/60g tuna fish with cooked pasta spirals, mixed with a
little vinaigrette, watercress and lettuce)

MID-AFTERNOON
one round of cucumber or salad sandwiches
tea or coffee

EVENING MEAL
cheese salad
(a colourful mixed salad from red and green peppers,
sweetcorn, grated carrot, lettuce and tomatoes, watercress,
etc. Add 1oz/30g grated cheese from allowance)
two boiled potatoes
OR
SALMON FISHCAKES (p.135)

SUPPER
one portion porridge
one apple, a few grapes

**Please do not forget your water intake today and
every day. Drink water between mouthfuls, and sip
water during the day at every opportunity.**

5 DAYS TO A FLATTER STOMACH

DAY 3

BREAKFAST
one portion of porridge or Rice Crispies
tea or decaffeinated coffee

MID-MORNING
one slice of toast or one muffin with butter and 1 tsp jam
OR
half a baguette or slice of crusty French bread, with butter
and 1 tsp jam

LUNCH
SPANISH OMELETTE (p.142) with green salad and either a
jacket potato or handful of chips
OR
one hardboiled egg, sliced, on two 'original' Ryvitas, spread
with ¹/₂ tsp MAYONNAISE (p.157)

MID-AFTERNOON
sliced apple and banana mixed

EVENING MEAL
BEEF GOULASH (p.126) with broccoli spears and rice
OR
KEDGEREE (p.132) with mixed salad
OR
BAKED BEANS (p.135) or MUSHROOMS ON TOAST (p.156)
one MERINGUE (p.154) filled with sliced strawberries or fresh
raspberries
OR
BANANA AND STRAWBERRY MOUSSE (p.153)

SUPPER
one Weetabix or Shredded Wheat
¹/₄ pint/150ml skimmed milk
sultanas and flaked almonds

DAY 4

BREAKFAST
Rice Crispies
one boiled egg with slice of toast
4fl oz/100ml glass fresh orange juice

MID-MORNING
one MERINGUE (p.149) filled with 2 tsp fromage frais

LUNCH
2oz/60g boiled pasta with one slice ham, cut in strips, with
grated Parmesan cheese
OR
8oz/250g mashed potatoes, one slice ham, lettuce, carrot
OR
cottage cheese salad
(3$\frac{1}{2}$oz/100g cottage cheese, lettuce, chives, pineapple chunks,
celery, chopped peppers and half an avocado [optional])

MID-AFTERNOON
one banana or sliced apple
tea or coffee
glass of water

EVENING MEAL
COD AND PRAWN PIE (p.134)
OR
VEGETABLE PAELLA (p.141)
OR
CORONATION CHICKEN (p.131)

one sliced pear with 1tbsp CHOCOLATE SAUCE (p.158)

SUPPER
one slice of wholemeal toast
butter and jam

DAY 5

BREAKFAST
stay with porridge if you love it, otherwise
Rice Crispies
OR
one egg, scrambled on one slice toast
4fl oz/100ml glass fresh orange juice

MID-MORNING
bio-yoghurt with a sliced banana
OR
one piece of cake from list (p.148)

LUNCH
mushrooms (p.156) or cheese on toast (p.155)
OR
sandwich made with either 2oz/50g cottage cheese, three to
four sliced grapes or mixed salad, and unbleached white bread

MID-AFTERNOON
one round of thinly sliced cucumber OR tomato sandwiches

EVENING MEAL
GRILLED SALMON WITH TARRAGON BUTTER (p.133)
three boiled potatoes
2 tbsp asparagus or French beans
OR
CHEESE SOUFFLÉ (p.143) with a green salad
OR
roast chicken breast
two roast potatoes
2 tbsp puréed carrots, sprouts and cauliflower
gravy
stuffing

RICE PUDDING (p.152) OR HOT FRUIT MERINGUE (p.154)

5 DAYS TO A FLATTER STOMACH

SUPPER
1oz/30g bran flakes with 4fl oz/100ml skimmed milk
and a sliced apple

. . . AND FINALLY

What if you've got just a day or so to look your very best? What if you've suddenly been invited somewhere and want to wear your slinkiest outfit or most figure-hugging skirt? Do you spend all day nibbling bits of fruit?

This isn't a weight-loss diet, but when a flatter stomach is very important to you it's easy to fall into the trap of eating nothing the day before, or snacking on raw vegetables. This isn't the right approach. So what do you do?

1. Start the day before if you can, and for supper have a stir-fry with plenty of sweetcorn, peas and other fresh vegetables. Drink two or three glasses of water during the evening whether you like it or not and have 1½oz/40g of All Bran or bran flakes for supper, with a few grapes, sliced apple and an orange if possible
2. For breakfast on the day itself, eat one slice of unbleached white toast
3. Make a round of sandwiches, either tuna fish, cottage cheese or jam, and cut into four. Eat one every hour, with a glass of water which has an orange slice in it
4. For lunch, have a banana topped with a carton of live natural yoghurt
5. Two hours later, have either half an avocado pear eaten from its shell, or another banana, and drink a glass of skimmed milk slowly
6. About 4pm, have a jacket potato, or 6oz/180g mashed potato, water, or cold potato salad if you are at work. (6oz/180g potato, cubed, with 1tsp mayonnaise)
7. About 6pm eat a carton of rice pudding slowly

DO NOT EAT AFTER THIS

This regime works extremely well for just one day, after which you must go back to normal eating.

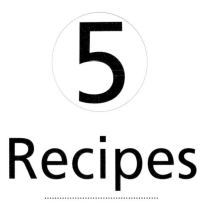

Recipes

I stated at the very beginning of this book that I didn't want to put temptation in your way by including too many meal suggestions that would have you chained to the cooker for hours. I have restricted the number of options because there should be enough variety in these recipes to suit every taste.

Stay with the exact suggestions on the standard 5-day plan. For The Maintenance Plan, feel free to mix and match the recipes. You will find that there are some recipes not specifically given in the diet.

There are five of everything. The categories are:

1. Beef	**5. Vegetarian**	**9. Snacks and**	**10. Sauces**
2. Chicken	**6. Salads**	**their calorie**	**and their**
3. Fish	**7. Cakes**	**contents**	**dressings**
4. Pasta	**8. Puddings**		

I won't sacrifice quality just because this is a diet. I have stoically stood by natural fats, like butter and cream, and I will not touch the pumped-up artificial alternatives labelled low-fat. The quantities are carefully controlled in any event.

Feel free to play around with quantities to suit your own requirements. I have taken care to include meals which are favourites with most people, including children. Each recipe states clearly how many people it will feed.

FIVE BEEF RECIPES

These five beef recipes should find favour with most tastes:

1. **Spaghetti bolognaise**
2. **Shepherd's pie**
3. **Chilli con carne**
4. **Beef goulash**
5. **Beef stroganoff**

The quantities given are for two portions. If you are a family of three or four, simply increase quantities accordingly.

SPAGHETTI BOLOGNAISE

Serves 2   Calories per portion – 383

8oz/250g extra lean mince	8oz/250g fresh spaghetti
1¹/₂ tbsp olive oil	few leaves fresh oregano or ¹/₂ tsp dried oregano
1 small onion, finely chopped	
1 clove garlic, crushed (*optional*)	salt and freshly ground black pepper
8oz/250g tinned chopped tomatoes with herbs	green salad
1 tbsp concentrated tomato paste	Parmesan cheese

1. In a large frying-pan, fry the mince without any added fat or oil until any fat runs clear. Drain. Set the meat aside.
2. Heat the oil and gently sauté the onion until softened. Drain excess oil.
3. Add the mince, garlic, tomatoes and tomato paste. Turn down the heat, cover pan and simmer for 5 minutes.
4. Add the spaghetti to the boiling water and cook as directed on the packet.
5. Add the oregano to the mince mixture. Stir.
6. Check seasoning and add salt and pepper if necessary. Drain the pasta, add the mince mixture to the pasta and toss.
7. Serve with a green salad and a sprinkling of Parmesan cheese.

SHEPHERD'S PIE

Serves 2   Calories per portion – 283

8oz/250g lean mince	¼oz/7g butter
1 Oxo cube	2fl oz/50ml skimmed milk
8oz/250g potatoes, peeled and sliced	1 tbsp gravy powder
1 small onion, finely chopped	salt and freshly ground black pepper
4 carrots, finely chopped	

1. Preheat the oven to 180°C/350°F/Gas mark 4.

2. In a large frying-pan, fry the mince without added fat or oil until any fat runs clear. Drain and put the mince in a large saucepan.

3. Add the stock cube, dissolve as directed and leave to simmer for 10 minutes.

4. Boil the potatoes until soft.

5. Add the onion and carrots to the mince.

6. When the potatoes are done, drain and mash with the butter and milk. Leave to cool slightly.

7. In a cup, mix the gravy powder with a little water until smooth. Add to the mince, stirring all the time. Put the mince in an ovenproof dish, season to taste and top with the mashed potato.

8. Place in the preheated oven until brown on top. Serve with green vegetables.

CHILLI CON CARNE

Serves 2   Calories per portion – 392

This recipe is made exactly as the one for spaghetti bolognaise, but instead of adding oregano, use either one finely chopped chilli pepper, or 1–2 tsp chilli powder (depending on how hot you like your food). Cook 4oz/125g of rice instead of pasta.

BEEF GOULASH

Serves 2   Calories per portion – 319 without rice, 429 with 3oz/90g rice

2 tsp olive oil	4 sliced mushrooms
8oz/250g best stewing steak	1 tsp paprika
1 small onion, chopped	salt and freshly ground black pepper
1 Oxo cube	
1 glass red wine	*crème fraîche*
½ red pepper, chopped	
2–3 chopped tomatoes or one small tin chopped tomatoes	

1. Put 2 tsp of olive oil into a frying-pan and add the steak.
2. Preheat the oven to 160°C/300°F/Gas mark 3.
3. Brown the meat on all sides. Add the onion.
4. Dissolve the Oxo cube in a little water. Add to the meat.
5. Pour the mixture into a casserole dish, add the wine, red pepper, tomatoes and mushrooms.
6. Cook slowly for about 2½ hours, stirring occasionally.
7. Add the paprika and season to taste.
8. Boil the rice according to directions on packet, or prepare potatoes and vegetables. Just before serving and when casserole has cooled slightly, add the *crème fraîche* and stir.

BEEF STROGANOFF

Serves 2   Calories per portion – approximately 459

3¹/₂oz/100g rice	black peppercorns, crushed
1 tbsp olive oil	salt
1 small onion, chopped	1–2 tsp paprika, to taste
clove garlic, chopped (*optional*)	4oz/125g mushrooms, chopped
8oz/250g fillet or sirloin steak, cut into strips OR 8oz/250g specially prepared beef stir-fry strips	1 tbsp brandy (*optional*)
	2 tbsp *crème fraîche*
1 red pepper, cut into strips	

1. Boil the rice according to directions on the packet.
2. Heat the oil in a large frying-pan. Add the onion, garlic and sauté gently until transparent.
3. Add the beef and turn on a high heat to seal on all sides.
4. Turn down the heat and cook for another minute. Add the red pepper strips, peppercorns, salt, paprika and mushrooms.
5. Turn the heat up high, add the brandy and flambé. Remove from heat and stir in the *crème fraîche.*
6. Serve immediately on the boiled rice with a green salad.

FIVE CHICKEN RECIPES

Chicken is wonderful for slimming because it has very little fat, is full of nutrients and can be used as the base for a wide variety of recipes. It has the added bonus of being quick to prepare and cook, and has only 42 calories per ounce (147 calories per 100g) roasted. The average portion would be 3–4oz/90–125g.

Chicken should always be cooked through thoroughly, not pink in the centre. Once cooked, cool the chicken speedily. **Never** leave chicken lying about as it can become a breeding ground for bacteria.

These are your five chicken choices:
1. **Stir-fried chicken with vegetables**
2. **Cajun chicken**
3. **Tarragon chicken**
4. **Coronation chicken**
5. **Spicy yoghurt-baked chicken**

An obvious choice is plain roast chicken with vegetables. All these recipes call for skinless, boneless chicken breasts. Either buy ready-packed, or do it yourself.

BASIC CHICKEN BREAST PREPARATION
Serves 1   Calories per portion – approximately 154

1 average-sized chicken breast	1–2 tbsp vegetable or olive oil

1. Trim off any excess fat or skin from the chicken breast and slice the breast into thin strips.
2. In a frying-pan, heat the oil gently on a low heat and add the chicken.
3. Turn the chicken quickly, sealing all sides, until the strips are white in colour. Turn down the heat, cover the pan and allow to cook through. This should take 8–10 minutes.
4. Allow to brown slightly, without burning.
5. Drain off excess oil by turning chicken out on to piece of

You now have the basis for a whole range of different tastes. I suggest you also try adding: chopped lemon grass and garlic for Thai-style chicken; cumin and coriander for a stronger curried taste; or chopped tomatoes, garlic and oregano for an Italian flavour.

STANDARD STIR-FRIED CHICKEN WITH VEGETABLES

Serves 1   Calories per portion – 198

1 chicken breast	soy sauce, to taste
bought stir-fry vegetable mixture OR bean sprouts, tinned waterchestnuts, mushrooms, mangetouts, chinese leaf, small broccoli florets and baby sweetcorn	lemon pepper, to taste
	dried red chillies, to taste

1. Prepare the chicken as for Basic Chicken Breast (p.128).
2. Add either the bought stir-fry vegetable mixture or your own mixture.
3. Toss the vegetables on a high heat for about 1–2 minutes, no longer. The mixture can easily turn into a 'stew' which is not so pleasant.
4. Add a good dash of soy sauce and a sprinkling of lemon pepper and dried chillies. Serve immediately.

CAJUN CHICKEN

Serves 1   Calories per portion – 253 with rice, 154 with salad

This is a variation on the Standard Stir-fried Chicken. Keep the chicken breast whole and make up a crunchy coating.

1 tsp citrus pepper, ground	1 tsp dried red chillies, ground
1 tsp coriander seeds, ground	1 chicken breast
1 tsp cayenne pepper, ground	butter
1 tsp dried garlic granules, ground	1–2 tbsp olive oil
1 tsp dried onion granules, ground	50g rice or selection of salad leaves

1. Combine the herbs and spices.

2. Lightly brush the chicken with melted butter. Press into the herbs and spice mixture. Cover all surfaces.

3. Heat the oil in a frying-pan. Add the chicken and sauté gently until cooked thoroughly (about 5–8 minutes depending on the thickness of the chicken). Turn up the heat and sear until nearly blackened.

4. Serve immediately on either a bed of rice, or salad leaves, scoring the chicken diagonally for presentation.

TARRAGON CHICKEN

Serves 1   Calories per portion – 353 with pasta, 244 as a salad

1 chicken breast	salt and freshly ground black pepper
2oz/60g pasta spirals or *penne*, preferably fresh	
	1tbsp *crème fraîche*
1oz/30g mushrooms sliced	salad leaves
handful fresh taragon or ¹/₂ tsp dried taragon	

1. Prepare Basic Chicken Breast (p.128).

2. Meanwhile, boil the pasta according to the directions on the packet.

3. Add the mushrooms and tarragon to the chicken. Season according to taste.

4. When ready (the chicken should be white throughout with no hint of pink flesh), take off the heat and add the *crème fraîche*. Stir and serve immediately. *Do not allow the mixture to cook any further as it will separate and become greasy.*

5. Drain the pasta and serve immediately with a garnish of watercress and other green salad leaves, or omit the pasta and serve on a bed of salad leaves with a little vinaigrette.

For Pesto Chicken, simply substitute basil for the tarragon and add 1 tsp of pesto sauce.

CORONATION CHICKEN

Serves 1 Calories per portion – 232, 351 with rice

1oz/30g (dry weight) basmati rice	few flaked almonds (*optional*)
1 tsp apricot jam	1 small chicken breast (6oz/150g), roasted, cooled and cut into strips
1/2 tbsp mayonnaise	
1–2 tsp curry powder	mixed salad leaves (*optional*)

1. Set the rice to boil.

2. Mix the jam, mayonnaise, curry powder, almonds and chicken. Combine thoroughly. Add more curry powder if you like it spicy.

3. Drain the rice, cool and arrange on a plate with the chicken mixture.

4. Alternatively, serve on a bed of mixed salad leaves and omit the rice.

SPICY YOGHURT-BAKED CHICKEN

Serves 2 Calories per portion – approximately 275

1 carton plain live bio-yoghurt	1 clove garlic, crushed (*optional*)
juice of 1 fresh lime	2 chicken breasts
a little fresh ginger root, grated	4oz/125g basmati rice
few fennel seeds	green salad
1 tsp each cumin, turmeric and cayenne pepper	

1. To prepare the marinade, combine the yoghurt, lime juice, spices and garlic in a bowl and mix thoroughly.

2. Place the chicken in the marinade, coat completely, cover and set aside for 2–8 hours.

3. Preheat the oven at 180°C/350°F/Gas mark 4.

4. Place chicken in an ovenproof dish and cook in the oven for about 25 minutes. Spread the marinade over the chicken and return to the oven uncovered, for about 30 minutes.

5. Boil the rice as directed on the packet, drain, add the chicken and serve with a green salad.

FIVE FISH RECIPES

Here are your five fish choices:

1. Kedgeree
2. Poached or grilled fillet of salmon or cod
3. Cod and prawn pie
4. Salmon fishcakes
5. Scampi Provençale

KEDGEREE

Serves 2   Calories per portion – approximately 390

Served as a main meal with a green salad or other vegetables, this makes a slightly exotic, very nourishing and tasty meal. Alternatively, served as a light lunch dish, or traditionally as a breakfast dish, you can halve the quantities given here. Better still, train yourself to eat less, try having half now and half later.

2 fillets smoked haddock, about 8oz/250g each	1 tsp turmeric
skimmed milk to poach	pinch each cayenne pepper and nutmeg
3¹/₂oz/100g basmati rice	2 hard-boiled eggs, shelled and cut into quarters
¹/₄oz/7g butter	
¹/₂ an onion, finely chopped	salt and freshly ground black pepper
1–2 tsp mild curry powder	

1. Place the haddock in an ovenproof dish or large frying-pan, cover with the milk and set to poach gently until softened through (about 8 minutes).
2. Meanwhile, boil the rice in enough water to cover, following directions on the packet. When cooked, drain thoroughly.
3. Melt the butter in another frying-pan and gently fry the onion until soft.
4. Add the drained rice, curry powder, turmeric, cayenne pepper and nutmeg to the onion. Stir.
5. Remove the haddock when cooked and flake the fish, reserving the cooking milk. Add the fish to the rice mixture.
6. Add the eggs and milk to the rice and fish mixture.
7. Season if necessary, stir and serve hot.

POACHED, BAKED OR GRILLED FILLET OF SALMON OR COD

Serves 1   Calories per oz/30g – salmon 51, cod 23

If you cook two salmon fillets, you can reserve one fillet for lunch. If you don't have salmon, poach the cod in a little milk and serve with the potatoes and some runner beans or green salad. Cold cod isn't very appetizing, so you can substitute tuna for cold salmon.

1 salmon fillet, 4–6oz/125–180g or 1 cod fillet, 4–6oz/125–180g	**2 tbsp french beans**
	1 tsp butter
2 potatoes	**fresh tarragon leaves, chopped or a pinch of dried tarragon**
2 tbsp carrots	

1. Poach, bake or grill the fish:

To poach the fish – place the fish in a lidded frying-pan with ¹/₂in/1cm of water, just enough to cover the bottom. Poach gently for about eight minutes, or until cooked through.

To bake the fish – preheat oven to 180°C/350°F/Gas mark 4. Place the fish in a covered container and bake in the oven for about 20 minutes.

To grill the fish – grill with a dot of butter.

2. Set the potatoes and carrots to boil.

3. When the fish is nearly ready, put the beans on to boil or steam for about three minutes.

4. Soften the butter and combine with the tarragon.

5. Drain the fish if poaching and top with the tarragon butter. Add the potatoes, garnish with parsley and serve immediately with the vegetables.

COD AND PRAWN PIE

Serves 2   Calories per portion – 495

³/₄ pint/360ml skimmed milk	1 tsp mustard powder
8oz/250g cod fillet or two frozen portions, thawed	salt and freshly ground black pepper
1lb/50g old potatoes, peeled and diced	sprig of fresh parsley, chopped
handful of broccoli florets, broken into small pieces	2oz/60g Cheddar cheese
	4oz/125g frozen prawns, thawed and drained
1oz/30g cornflour	

1. Put half the milk into a small frying-pan and add the cod, whole. Cover and bring to a gentle simmer on a very low heat. Poach gently until cooked in the middle (about 8–10 minutes). Drain and reserve the liquid.

2. Break the fish into large chunks or flakes and put into a shallow ovenproof casserole dish. Preheat the oven to 180°C/350°F/Gas mark 4.

3. Boil the potatoes.

4. Boil or steam the broccoli for 3 minutes. Drain and reserve.

5. Make the sauce by putting the reserved milk into a saucepan and heating gently. Mix the cornflour with a tablespoon of milk until it forms a smooth paste. Add the paste to the milk in the pan and raise the heat slightly, stirring constantly as the mixture thickens, to avoid burning or lumps forming.

6. Take off the heat. Add the mustard powder, seasoning and parsley.

7. Stir in the cheese and beat gently as the cheese melts.

8. Drain the potatoes and mash with the remaining milk.

9. Arrange the broccoli over the cod chunks, add the prawns and pour on the cheese sauce.

10. Spoon the mashed potato over the top or pipe in swirls if you want a more dressy appearance.

11. Place in the oven for 20–30 minutes, or until the top is golden. Serve with fresh peas and carrots.

SALMON FISHCAKES

Serves 2 (2 fishcakes per person)   Calories per portion – 347

2 large potatoes (about 8oz/250g each)	**sprig of parsley, chopped**
8oz/250g salmon fillet	**juice and zest of $\frac{1}{2}$ a lemon**
1 small onion, or a few shallots, chopped	**$\frac{1}{4}$oz/7g butter**
salt and freshly ground black pepper	

1. Boil the potatoes for exactly 5 minutes. Drain and cool slightly.

2. Preheat the oven to 190°C/375°F/Gas mark 5.

3. Put the salmon and onion or shallots into a frying-pan, cover and poach for about 5 minutes in a little water until they are tender.

4. Drain and place in a bowl. Season and add the parsley.

5. Remove the skin from the potatoes. Grate each potato into the bowl containing the salmon mixture.

6. Mix the fish and potato together quite roughly, as the beauty of these fishcakes is their 'jumbled' appearance.

7. Using a zester if possible, grate the lemon into the mixture, then add half the squeezed lemon.

8. Grease a baking sheet with the butter, leaving a little to brush over the tops of the fishcakes. Form the fish mixture into small balls and gently flatten them out on the sheet. Brush the tops with melted butter. Cook in the preheated oven for 10–15 minutes or until golden on top. Turn once.

SCAMPI PROVENÇALE

Serves 2   Calories per portion – 204 without rice, 274 with rice

¹/₂ a medium onion, chopped	14oz/400g tin chopped tomatoes with herbs
1 clove garlic, crushed	
8oz/250g raw scampi or very large prawns	salt and freshly ground black pepper
small glass of dry white wine	4oz/125g rice or a green salad
1 small chilli, chopped	

1. Heat the oil in a non-stick frying-pan. Add the onion and garlic and sauté until soft. Remove and set aside.

2. Add the scampi or prawns to the oil and cook over a medium heat for 1–2 minutes. Remove and set aside.

3. Return the onion and garlic to the pan, add the wine, chilli, tomatoes and seasoning. Simmer for fifteen minutes.

4. Add the scampi or prawns and heat through.

5. Serve garnished with parsley on a bed of boiled rice or a green salad.

FIVE PASTA RECIPES

You simply cannot beat pasta for versatility. Low in fat and high in starch and protein, pasta is one of the best foods for any slimming diet and you should try to eat a portion several times a week. Even plain boiled pasta with a little melted butter and cheese tastes marvellous!

Many of your chicken and beef recipes also contain pasta as an accompanying ingredient, but these dishes concentrate on pasta as the main body of the dish.

1. **Spaghetti with smoked salmon, dill and watercress**
2. **Spaghetti alla carbonara**
3. **Pasta spirals with lemon and dill**
4. **Pasta primavera**
5. **Peppered salmon or cod with pasta and salad**

SPAGHETTI WITH SMOKED SALMON, DILL AND WATERCRESS

Serves 2   Calories per portion – 236

4oz/125g fresh spaghetti	1 bunch watercress, washed and stripped into leaves
1 tsp olive oil or ¹/₂oz/7g butter	
1 clove garlic, crushed (*optional*)	salt and freshly ground black pepper
1oz/30g smoked salmon, cut into thin strips	

1. Cook the spaghetti in 2 pints/1.25ml of water for three minutes. Drain.
2. Heat the oil or butter in a large frying-pan. Add the garlic, salmon and watercress, and cook for thirty seconds, stirring constantly.
3. Add the spaghetti to the pan, season to taste, heat through and serve immediately.

SPAGHETTI ALLA CARBONARA

Serves 2   Calories per portion – 260

I first experienced this dish in 1970 when staying with an Italian friend in her cramped bedsit in London. With only a single gas ring to cook on, she showed me how to conjure up this magnificent dish in twenty minutes, which is now reduced to ten minutes due to the widespread availability of fresh pasta. I have adapted it slightly for slimming purposes, but remember that we eat smaller portions anyway!

2 rashers smoked back bacon	coarsely ground black pepper
3¹/₂oz/100g fresh spaghetti	2 tbsp single cream
1 egg yolk	a splash of good olive oil

1. Using a standard sauce or frying-pan, fry the bacon without fat until well cooked. Set aside.

2. Fill the pan with 1 pint/600ml of water, bring to the boil and add the spaghetti.

3. While the spaghetti is cooking, chop the bacon into pieces, and mix the egg yolk, pepper and cream in a cup.

4. After three minutes, drain the spaghetti thoroughly and return to the pan, keeping the heat low. Add the olive oil, bacon bits, egg and cream mixture and toss.

5. Turn off the heat and continue stirring. (If you leave the heat on the eggs start to scramble.)

6. Serve immediately on a very hot plate.

PASTA WITH LEMON AND DILL

Serves 1   Calories per portion – 198

2fl oz/50ml milk	pinch of salt
2 tbsp freshly squeezed lemon juice	2oz/60g fresh pasta spirals
	tiny pat of butter
1 thin strip lemon rind about 2in/5cm long	1 tsp finely cut fresh dill OR 1 tsp dried dill
1 tsp caraway seeds (*optional*)	

1. Put the milk, lemon juice, lemon rind, caraway seeds and salt into a large saucepan.
2. Bring to the boil, reduce the liquid and simmer for three minutes.
3. Add the spirals and enough cold water to cover.
4. Simmer for three minutes until the pasta is cooked. Drain.
5. Discard the lemon rind, stir in the butter and the dill. Serve immediately.

PASTA PRIMAVERA

Serves 1   Calories per portion – 278

2oz/60g fresh pasta spirals or penne	1 tsp pesto sauce
	2 tsp *crème fraîche*
1tbsp olive oil	salt and freshly ground black pepper
handful of mangetouts, baby sweetcorn, sugar-snap peas, carrot sticks, red and green peppers, been sprouts	

1. Cook the pasta until soft. Drain and keep warm.
2. In a deep frying-pan or wok, heat the oil and add the mixed vegetables. Toss on a high heat for one minute.
3. Add the drained pasta and the pesto sauce. Turn for thirty seconds.
4. Remove from heat, add the *crème fraîche*, stir, check seasoning and serve immediately.

PEPPERED SALMON OR COD

Serves 2   Calories per portion – approximately 206

This dish is terribly easy to make.

3¹/₂oz/100g pasta spirals	citrus pepper (you can buy this in jars in most supermarkets)
selection of salad leaves	
1 salmon fillet or 1 cod fillet, cut into chunks or strips	a little lemon juice
	chopped fresh parsley
¹/₄oz/7g butter or oil	

1. Cook the pasta according to instructions on packet. Drain and keep warm.
2. Arrange some salad leaves on a plate.
3. Place the fish chunks on a flat plate and brush with a little melted butter or oil, so that the citrus pepper will stick when coated.
4. Sprinkle the fish liberally with the citrus pepper, turning until all the surfaces are covered. Press in firmly so that none of the coating falls off.
5. Heat the butter in a frying-pan and add the fish, cooking gently for three minutes on each side. Turn it carefully to avoid breaking the flesh.
6. Turn up the heat and fry for another thirty seconds until slightly blackened and crisp.
7. Add the pasta to the pan. Toss for a few seconds and turn on to the bed of salad leaves. Sprinkle with a little lemon juice and chopped parsley.

FIVE VEGETARIAN RECIPES

Many of the recipes I have already recommended to you are adaptable for vegetarians, especially some of the pasta and stir-fry dishes.

Here are five further popular recipes:

1. **Vegetable paella**
2. **Spanish or herb omelette**
3. **Baby Balti vegetables**
4. **Cheese soufflé**
5. **Mushroom stroganoff**

VEGETABLE PAELLA

Serves 2   Calories per portion – 180

$^{1}/_{2}$ an aubergine, chopped	1 clove garlic, crushed
salt	$3^{1}/_{2}$oz/100g long-grain rice
1 tbsp olive oil	1 small tin of chopped tomatoes with herbs
$^{1}/_{2}$ a small onion, chopped	$^{1}/_{2}$ tsp turmeric
3 slices red and green pepper, chopped	coarsely ground black pepper
$^{1}/_{2}$ a carrot, chopped	fresh parsley

1. Lay the aubergine on a board and cover with salt. Leave for twenty minutes. Wash and drain.
2. Heat the olive oil in a large frying-pan, add the onion and gently sauté until soft.
3. Add the peppers, aubergine, carrot and garlic, and stir. Add the raw rice.
4. Add the tomatoes, plus $^{1}/_{2}$ pint/300ml of water and the turmeric. Season to taste.
5. Bring to the boil, then reduce heat and simmer until all the water has been absorbed by the rice.
6. Serve with a good sprinkling of parsley.

SPANISH OR HERB OMELETTE

Serves 1   Calories per portion – approximately 220–250

2 medium eggs	red and green pepper, onion, mushrooms, few chunks of cold potato all chopped (for the Spanish omelette)
salt and freshly ground coarse black pepper	
1/4oz/7g butter	
mixed herbs (for the herb omelette)	

1. Break the eggs into a bowl and beat them lightly. Season.
2. Put the butter into a medium frying-pan and heat until hot but not blackened.
3. Add the vegetables to the butter and stir together for one minute. Add the eggs and cook on the bottom only. Cook the top of the omelette by holding under a medium grill until set.

Herb omelette Add the eggs, covering the bottom of the pan quickly. Using a fork, draw the edges of the omelette into the centre letting the liquid run to the outside. Keep this up until the omelette is beginning to set but is still moist. Add the herbs, fold and serve immediately.

BABY BALTI VEGETABLES

Serves 2   Calories per portion – 132, with naan bread 213

There are a wide variety of baby vegetables available these days, usually aimed at the stir-fry market. This simple recipe can be prepared in a very short space of time, with little equipment.

8 potatoes	4oz/125g chickpeas or 1 small tin
8 carrots	handful of mangetouts
6 baby courgettes	8 baby sweetcorn
2 tbsp corn oil	8 cherry tomatoes
8 baby onions	1 tsp dried chillies
1 tsp ginger paste	3/4 tbsp sesame seeds
1 tsp garlic purée	1 piece naan bread
1 tbsp chilli sauce	

1. Bring a pan of water to the boil and add the potatoes and the carrots.

2. After 5–8 minutes (depending on the size of the vegetables), add the courgettes and boil for a further two minutes. Drain and reserve.

3. Heat the oil in a large frying-pan or wok. Add the onions and fry until golden brown.

4. Lower the heat and add the ginger paste, garlic purée and chilli sauce.

5. Add the chickpeas and stir-fry over a medium heat until all the moisture has been absorbed.

6. Add the cooked potatoes, carrots and courgettes, plus the mangetouts, baby sweetcorn and tomatoes. Stir over the heat for a further 2 minutes.

7. Add the crushed chillies, turn on to a serving plate and sprinkle with the sesame seeds. Serve with naan bread.

CHEESE SOUFFLÉ

Serves 2   Calories per portion – approximately 328

Soufflés are not nearly as difficult or exacting to make as people think, and I have often guessed at the quantities, thrown them all in and still had a sensational result.

¹/₂oz/15g self-raising flour	¹/₂oz/15g fresh grated Parmesan cheese (*optional*)
¹/₄ pint/150ml skimmed milk	
¹/₄oz/7g butter	salt and freshly ground black pepper
3 large eggs, separated (you will only use 2 yolks and 3 whites)	green salad
2oz/60g strong Cheddar, Leicester or Cheshire cheese, finely grated	

1. Preheat your oven to 200°C/400°F/Gas mark 6.

2. Butter a medium soufflé dish and tie a piece of greaseproof paper round the outside to hold the soufflé as it rises.

3. In a saucepan, mix the flour with a little cold milk to form a smooth paste. Gently bring to a simmer, adding the rest of the milk, stirring all the time as it thickens. Add the butter.

4. Allow the sauce to cool slightly, making sure that it does not form a skin over the top by covering the pan.
5. Add the two egg yolks and beat the mixture until it is smooth.
6. Add the cheese and seasoning.
7. Whisk the three egg whites until stiff but not dry. Add the cheese and sauce mixture to the egg whites not the other way round. Transfer immediately to the soufflé dish and bake for about 15–20 minutes, or until golden brown on top. Eat immediately with a green salad.

MUSHROOM STROGANOFF

Serves 1   Calories per portion – 316

3oz/90g rice (1oz/30g raw weight)	1 tbsp *crème fraîche*
	1 tsp tomato purée
½oz/15g butter	salt, nutmeg, freshly ground black pepper
½ a small onion, finely chopped	
garlic, crushed (*optional*)	paprika to garnish
8oz/250g mushrooms (a variety if possible)	

1. Boil the rice until cooked (follow directions on packet).
2. Melt the butter in a very large frying-pan. Add the onion and garlic, and cook until transparent, about five minutes.
3. Add the mushrooms (they will seem a lot but they reduce in size). Keep stirring until most of the liquid has evaporated.
4. Stir in the *crème fraîche* and tomato purée. Add seasonings to taste and cook for a further 2–3 minutes. Top with paprika and serve on a bed of rice.

FIVE SUMMER AND WINTER SALADS

These salads can be eaten as an accompaniment to a main meal, or as a meal on their own:

1. Caesar Salad

2. Waldorf Salad

3. Winter Salad

4. Greek Pasta Salad

5. Courgette, Carrot, Grapefruit and Avocado Salad

CAESAR SALAD

Serves 2   Calories per large bowl – approximately 120

home-made mayonnaise (p.157)	vegetable oil
garlic clove, crushed	1oz/30g Parmesan cheese, coarsely grated
1 Cos lettuce	
1 large slice thick-cut stale bread	

1. Make the mayonnaise as directed. Add the garlic.

2. Wash and dry the Cos lettuce and separate into leaves

3. Make the croûtons by cutting the bread into half-inch cubes. Heat the oil until very hot and fry the cubes quickly until golden brown, which will take a couple of minutes. Remove with a slotted spoon and blot dry.

4. Add the cooled croûtons to the lettuce bed. Add a tablespoon of the mayonnaise and toss together. Grate the Parmesan cheese liberally over the salad and serve.

WALDORF SALAD

Serves 2   Calories per portion – approximately 200

1 tbsp home-made mayonnaise (p.157)	20 grapes
1 red apple, sliced	12 walnuts
2 celery sticks, cut into ¹/₂in/1cm strips	lettuce

1. Make mayonnaise as directed.
2. Place the apple and celery in a bowl.
3. Add the grapes and walnuts. Bind with the mayonnaise and mix well.
4. Turn out on to the bed of lettuce and serve.

WINTER SALAD

Serves 2–3   Calories per portion – 138

¹/₄ of a white cabbage, shredded	10 dried, pre-soaked apricots, cut into small pieces
¹/₄ of a red cabbage, shredded	¹/₂oz/15g sultanas
2 carrots cut into julienne strips	¹/₂oz/15g sunflower seeds
¹/₂oz/15g flaked almonds	

NUT OIL DRESSING
Calories per portion – 30

1 clove garlic, crushed (*optional*)	2 tbsp hazelnut oil
2 tbsp white wine vinegar	salt and coarsely ground black pepper
2 tbsp virgin olive oil	
2 tbsp walnut oil	

1. Mix all the dry ingredients in a large bowl.
2. To make the dressing, mix together all the ingredients in a screw-top jar and shake well. Pour a small amount over the salad and toss until all the vegetables are evenly coated and glossy. *You do not have to use all the dressing*, it will keep.

GREEK PASTA SALAD

Serves 2   Calories per portion – 242

3¹/₂oz/100g pasta spirals	1 tsp capers
3/₂oz/100g feta cheese, cubed	8 pitted black olives
few strips each of red, green and yellow pepper	salad leaves
2 salad spring onions, sliced	

DRESSING

1 tbsp mayonnaise (p.157)	2 tbsp vinaigrette dressing (p.157)

1. Cook the pasta in boiling water according to the instructions on the packet.
2. Mix together the feta cheese, peppers and spring onions.
3. Drain and cool the pasta, add to the other ingredients and combine.
4. Sprinkle on the capers and olives and serve on a bed of salad leaves.
5. Mix the mayonnaise with the vinaigrette dressing until you have a creamy liquid. Pour over the salad and toss.

COURGETTE, CARROT, GRAPEFRUIT AND AVOCADO SALAD

Serves 2   Calories per portion – approximately 160

1 avocado	one grapefruit
1–2 carrots, scraped	vinaigrette dressing (p.157)
2 large courgettes	coarsely ground black pepper

1. Cut the avocado in two and discard the stone. Cut away the outer shell and slice each half into strips.
2. Using a potato peeler, slice long strips down the length of the carrots and courgettes, making ribbons.
3. Cut the grapefruit in two halves and using a grapefruit knife, carefully cut out segments. Add to the other vegetables.
4. Add enough vinaigrette dressing to coat the vegetables. Sprinkle with black pepper.

FIVE CAKE RECIPES

When you move on to The Maintenance Plan you can start to include some more puddings and cakes in your diet – as long as you can trust yourself to make a batch of cakes and not eat the lot!

I have selected just five cakes:

1. **Macaroons**
2. **Coconut pyramids**
3. **Meringues or walnut meringues**
4. **Date loaf**
5. **Whisked fatless sponge cake**

I have kept the amounts small so that you are not tempted, but if you have a family to bake for, double up on everything.

I make no apologies for the first three being unashamedly sugar treats, but as you are probably going to eat sugary treats from time to time, you may as well make them totally fat free, which is what all of these cakes are.

MACAROONS
Makes about 12   Calorie content – 78 per macaroon

4oz/125g caster sugar	12 split almonds for decoration, (*optional*)
2oz/60g ground almonds	
¹/₂ tbsp rice flour	rice paper
1 egg white	

1. Preheat your oven to 180°C/350°F/Gas mark 4.
2. In a bowl, mix the sugar, almonds and rice flour.
3. Beat the egg white lightly until fairly stiff but not dry, and add to the dry ingredients.
4. Beat the mixture to a smooth consistency, then form into small balls.
5. Line a baking sheet with the rice paper, place the balls on to it and add a split almond on each.
6. Cook for 20 minutes.
7. Cool, then cut round the rice paper, which is edible.

COCONUT PYRAMIDS

Makes about 12   Calorie content – 120 per pyramid

2 egg whites	1 tsp cornflour
5oz/150g caster sugar	rice paper
5oz/150g dessicated coconut	

1. Preheat the oven to 180°C/350°F/Gas mark 4.
2. Whisk the egg whites until stiff.
3. Fold in the sugar, coconut and cornflour.
4. Place small pyramids on a baking sheet lined with rice paper.
5. Bake for 8–10 minutes until crisp on the outside and slightly soft inside. Leave to cool, then cut round rice paper.

MERINGUES OR WALNUT MERINGUES

Makes about 11   Calories per meringue – 22 (plain) or 38 (walnut)

1 egg white	1oz/30g finely chopped walnuts
2oz/60g icing sugar	

1. Set the oven to 180°C/350°F/Gas mark 4.
2. Whisk the egg white until stiff.
3. Sift the icing sugar, and add to the egg white a spoonful at a time, continuing to whisk until very thick.
4. Carefully fold in the walnuts.
5. Place small moulds on a greased baking sheet and cook for 15–20 minutes. Transfer to a wire rack to cool and completely dry out before serving.

DATE LOAF

Makes one small 1lb (580g) loaf   Calories per slice – approximately 110

4oz/125g chopped and rolled dates	1 tsp mixed spice
	1 tsp cinnamon
6fl oz/170ml cold strong tea	2 tsp baking powder
4oz/125g wholewheat flour	1 small egg, beaten
3oz/90g soft brown sugar	demerara sugar for sprinkling

1. Put the dates into a bowl and cover with the cold tea. Leave for an hour to steep.

2. Preheat oven to 180°C/350°F/Gas mark 4.

3. Add the flour, sugar, spices, baking powder and the egg to the date mixture and mix thoroughly.

4. Turn into a lined and greased loaf tin and sprinkle the top with a little demerara sugar.

5. Bake for 1 hour, until cooked through. Leave in tin for five minutes, then turn on to a wire rack to cool.

WHISKED FATLESS SPONGE

Makes one small sponge with 8 slices   Calories about 152 per slice (with filling)

3 eggs	dash of vanilla essence or flavouring
4oz/125g caster sugar	
3oz/90g plain flour	2 tbsp warmed raspberry jam

1. Preheat oven to 190°C/375°F/Gas mark 5.

2. Line and grease two 9in/22.5cm sponge tins.

3. Using an electric beater, whisk together the eggs and sugar until very thick and pale in colour.

4. Fold in the sifted flour, a spoonful at a time, being careful not to beat. Add a dash of vanilla essence.

5. Divide the mixture between the two tins. Place in the oven for 30–40 minutes, or until the cakes spring back when lightly pressed.

6. Cool completely on a wire rack. Sandwich with warmed jam.

FIVE PUDDING RECIPES

1. Rice or semolina pudding
2. Pavlova and fresh fruit
3. Hot fruit meringues
4. Banana mousse and fruit snows
5. Winter fruit salad

RICE OR SEMOLINA PUDDING
Serves 3–4   Calories per serving – 147

I first became enthusiastic about milk puddings when I was pregnant with my second child during Christmas, and had to endure a long journey from the country to town and a freezing mile walk to the hospital for my check-ups. The whole procedure took half a day, but by starting with porridge and taking a pot of semolina with me I managed it with gusto – not easy when you're also trailing a two year old.

Since then I make either a semolina or rice pudding every week, summer or winter, because it is not only nourishing and healthy but it is equally as delicious hot or cold, especially the rice pudding. The calorie content is not at all high for a snack, and with the addition of stewed fruit or jam, you will have no need of another meal. Made with skimmed milk it's full of calcium, protein and starch. Try it!

1 pint/600ml skimmed milk	1½ tbsp sugar
2oz/60g semolina	

1. Set the oven to 180°C/350°F/Gas mark 4.
2. Put all the ingredients in a saucepan and boil, stirring.
3. When the mixture comes to the boil, turn down the heat and simmer for a few minutes, stirring to prevent the semolina becoming a sticky mass.
4. Pour into a lightly greased pudding basin and put in the oven for forty-five minutes.
5. Either eat straight away, hot, with a teaspoon of jam in the middle, or cool completely, pot into 3–4 empty yoghurt pots and refrigerate until needed. It can then be microwaved.

5 D A Y S T O A F L A T T E R S T O M A C H

RICE PUDDING

Quantities are as for the semolina pudding, but you do not have to heat through in a pan first. Use 2oz/60g short-grain (pudding) rice to 1 pint/600ml skimmed milk and place straight in moderate oven for two hours, or until cooked through. Stir occasionally to separate rice grains.

PAVLOVA AND FRESH FRUIT

Serves 2   Calories per portion – approximately 110

2 egg whites	a little whipped cream
2oz/60g caster sugar	
fresh strawberries or raspberries	

1. Whisk the egg whites until stiff in a clean mixing bowl.
2. Add the sugar a spoonful at a time, whisking until the mixture forms stiff peaks.
3. Form the mixture into two rounds on a greased, non-stick baking tray.
4. Bake in a medium-to-low oven for about thirty minutes, taking care not to brown the meringue.
5. Remove from oven and leave to cool and dry out completely.
6. Whisk the cream until stiff and add the fruit. Sandwich the two meringue rounds with the fruit and cream mixture.

N.B. *This sounds fattening because of the cream content, but you will be having only half the pudding, which is about 110 calories.*

BANANA AND STRAWBERRY MOUSSE AND FRUIT SNOWS

Serves 1   Calories per portion – 107

4oz/125g strawberries, fresh, frozen or tinned	1 medium or large banana

This can be eaten as either a dessert or a snack, but remember the high fibre content of the strawberries if you are susceptible to a delicate tummy! Place in a blender one medium or large banana (depending on your appetite), and 4oz/125g fresh or thawed frozen strawberries. Alternatively, use a tin of strawberries in fresh fruit juice (not syrup) which has been thoroughly drained, otherwise the mixture will be too liquid.

Blend for six seconds. Pour into a bowl and eat straight away. This mixture does keep for a few hours, but longer than that and it loses its 'fluffiness'.

FRUIT SNOW

Calories per portion – approximately 100, depending on the fruit

1 egg white	8oz/250g fruit purée
1oz/30g caster sugar	

This is an easy alternative for people who do not like the banana content of the mousse. I first made snows when my children were very small and would not eat fruit purées. I soon discovered that as long as their pudding was colourful and fluffy and served in a tall glass, they would eat it readily!

Stew any fruit down to a purée. It is especially good with apple and blackberries, strawberries or raspberries, rhubarb and gooseberries, and is handy for using up a glut of fruit you may have frozen since the summer.

Whisk one egg white until stiff, then fold in 1oz/30g caster sugar and whisk again until shiny and very stiff. Add about 8oz/250g of the fruit purée to the egg white *not the other way round*, fold together gently and serve immediately. This mixture makes enough for two or three servings, depending on how hungry you are, so if you are catering for larger numbers, increase accordingly.

HOT FRUIT MERINGUES

Serves 3–4   Calories per portion – 122

Hot fruit meringues are a simple way of serving a nice hot pudding in the winter without all the fuss of a pie or crumble, and certainly without all the calories!

Simply stew the available fruit in the usual way, making enough to fill a small ovenproof dish by two-thirds.

Although apple and blackberry, rhubarb or plain apple are the usual bases, I have also used combinations including banana and strawberry or apricot, prune and blackberry.

2 or 3 egg whites	stewed fruit
2oz/60g caster sugar	

Whisk two or three egg whites until stiff. Fold in 2oz/60g caster sugar and whisk again. Spoon over the cooled fruit mixture and use it to seal the edges of the dish to prevent the fruit 'boiling over'.

Bake in a medium oven 180°C/350°F/Gas mark 4, for about 10–15 minutes, or until golden brown on top. Serve.

WINTER FRUIT SALAD

Serves 2   Calories per portion – approximately 140

½ pint/300ml pure apple juice	4oz/125g blackberries
strip of orange zest	1 pear, sliced
1 cinnamon stick	1 tbsp brandy (*optional*)
a few cloves	1 tbsp *crème fraîche* or fromage frais
6oz/180g dried prunes, peaches and apricots, mixed	

1. Put the apple juice, orange zest, cinnamon stick, cloves and fruit into a pan and heat through on a very low heat until the mixture is simmering gently. Continue for 20 minutes, or until the fruit is soft.

2. Take the pan off the heat and stir in the brandy.

3. Either allow the salad to cool, or serve warm with a spoon of *crème fraîche* or fromage frais.

A GUIDE TO SNACKS

Not everybody likes fancy or spicy food, and not everybody can be bothered to even try cooking it. Well, it's just as easy to slim on a standard diet of good everyday foods such as toast, eggs and cheese, so here's a quick calorie guide to some of your favourites:

BEANS ON TOAST

Who on earth doesn't like beans on toast? Beans are very high in fibre (so if you have a problem with a bloated stomach I do not recommend them during the day), and do buy the normal type, not the low-sugar variety which is full of the chemical saccharine.

Use one slice of bread from a medium loaf, a scraping of butter from your allowance (3oz/90g a week or 2oz/60g for the 5-day plan) and half a tin of beans; depending on the make of beans you choose tin sizes vary. **Total calories will be about 200.**

POACHED EGG ON TOAST

A standard egg on a medium slice of toast with a scraping of butter comes to just **180 calories.**

SCRAMBLED EGGS ON TOAST

If you use the microwave to scramble your eggs you will need no extra butter to prevent sticking. Use two standard eggs, whisked with a splash of milk and serve on one lightly buttered slice of toast. **Total calories will be about 278.**

CHEESE ON TOAST

Using 1oz/30g of hard cheese such as Cheddar or Edam (calories vary as Edam is far less fatty than Cheddar) and one slice of bread, the calorie content will be **between 188 and 200.**

MUSHROOMS ON TOAST

Calories per serving – 193

Have you forgotten about mushrooms on toast? One of the simplest of snacks to make, and one of the most delicious in my opinion, people always exclaim in delight when you put this dish down in front of them on a cold night, or for a quick lunch.

You need a lot of mushrooms as they reduce greatly in volume whilst cooking. The portion size is about 8oz/250g per person.

Don't be alarmed by the cream and butter content. As with all dishes in this book, your portions are carefully controlled, and *crème fraîche* contains only 55 calories per level tablespoonful – the amount in this recipe.

Remember, there's absolutely no need to sacrifice taste and quality just because you're on a diet!

¹/₄oz/7g butter	one medium slice of bread
8oz/250g mushrooms (if you're feeling fancy, get a variety), sliced	1 tbsp *crème fraîche*
	paprika and some chopped parsley for serving
splash of milk	
salt and freshly ground coarse black pepper	

1. Heat the butter in a wide frying-pan until frothy.
2. Add the mushrooms, stir thoroughly and leave to cook. The mushrooms will produce some liquid.
3. Allow the liquid to evaporate, and add a splash of milk if the mushrooms look dry. Add seasoning to taste.
4. Toast the bread, and put on to a hot serving plate.
5. Just before serving, add the *crème fraîche* to the mushrooms. Top with a sprinkling of paprika and the parsley.

SAUCES AND DRESSINGS

FRENCH DRESSING OR VINAIGRETTE

The amount you make is up to you, depending on whether you are in a single household or are feeding half a dozen. The proportions are the same:

1. Use 3 parts olive oil or good vegetable oil to one part wine vinegar.
2. Pour into a screw-top jar.
3. Add 2 tsp Dijon mustard, 1 tsp sugar and some coarsely ground black pepper.
4. If you like garlic, add a crushed clove.
5. Shake the mixture thoroughly and taste. Adjust to suit your own tastes.

MAYONNAISE

Calories per dessertspoon – 40

Most people who are dieting worry unnecessarily about the high oil content in mayonnaise. The first consideration is that the fat content is good fat – not saturated – and the second is that we use tiny quantities. Use this mayonnaise on your hard-boiled eggs or your cold poached salmon. It will last for up to two days in the fridge. Use either a blender or an electric whisk for this.

1 egg yolk   **1 pint/600ml oil**

1. Separate one standard egg and reserve the white for something else (a meringue).
2. Use a good oil, and measure out about 1 pint/600ml.
3. Place the egg yolk in a clean bowl and add a few drops of oil, whisking all the time. Continue to add the oil by the drop until it seems that the mixture is amalgamating.
4. Graduate to letting the oil run in a thin stream. If you get tired and start to pour the oil too quickly, your impatience will be rewarded by the mixture curdling!
5. Continue until the mixture is thick and creamy.
6. If the mixture curdles try adding a spoonful of hot water or a small dash of vinegar. If you have spoilt it, however, start again with a fresh yolk and add the curdled mixture, bit by bit.

Now you have a basic mayonnaise – try a teaspoon of curry powder for curried mayonnaise (great for Coronation chicken p.131), or the grated zest of a lemon for lemon mayonnaise. Add some crushed garlic or finely chopped basil leaves.

FRESH CUSTARD
Calories – 80 per 5fl oz/150ml

Your own custard is so easy to make, I don't know why people don't make it more often.

1 egg yolk	**1 tsp cornflour**
1¹/₂ tbsp caster sugar	**¹/₂ pint/300ml skimmed milk**

1. Separate the egg and reserve the white for meringues.
2. In a small jug, mix the egg yolk with the sugar and corn-flour until it is a smooth paste. Add a little cold milk.
3. Put the rest of the milk in a pan and heat through. When it is coming to the boil, remove from the heat and add a little to the egg mixture, stirring all the time. Pour back into pan and keep heat low or the custard will curdle. Keep stirring while it thickens. Add a few drops of vanilla essence.

If the custard curdles, pour it into a cold bowl and whisk.

HOME-MADE CHOCOLATE SAUCE
Calories per heaped dessertspoon – 102

I don't use a lot of this, but a spoonful over half a tinned or baked pear makes a delicious and surprisingly low-calorie sweet dish. Don't make too much, or you'll be tempted to dip into it!

8oz/250g block dark plain chocolate	**2oz/60g caster sugar**
	3¹/₂fl oz/100ml double cream
12fl oz/350ml water	

1. Put the chocolate into the water, in a pan.
2. Add sugar. Bring to the boil and reduce to a simmer for 15 minutes.
3. Take from heat, stir in the cream. Refrigerate until needed.

The future – beating the bulge for good

Too many people will tell you that diets don't work. Of course they do. The people who usually say this are those who have either not found a diet which works for them, or who have failed in their attempts to re-educate their eating habits.

When someone says 'diet' you immediately think of cutting down on food, going for long periods feeling hungry and watching while everyone else eats the pudding and you have an apple. Well, I hope that by now you have realized that in my book, dieting simply means devising an eating regime which suits you, and not feeling that you have to rush out and do two hours of aerobics just because you ate a Walnut Whip. On the other hand, if you are a self-confessed glutton – and there's nothing wrong with that unless *you* are unhappy about it – you can't also hope to fit into size 10 clothes. There has to be a happy medium, and I hope I have supplied the key.

If there is one message which I want to give you for the future, it is to remember that *you* are in the driving seat when it comes to the beauty of your figure, and if you can conquer your fear of food you will never look back.

Never give up. Above all, I hope you have taken on board the fact that the keys to success are frequent eating and small portions. I'm still furious when I think of the hours I used to go without food, the appalling tiredness and lethargy I used to suffer, and the years I endured it, all in the name of being the same weight I am now. I now eat in the region of 2000 calories a day, feel brighter and healthier than I did twenty years ago and haven't gained a single pound! If you adopt my diet principles you will lose weight. You may start by gaining a few pounds as your metabolism takes a little time to adjust to your new diet, but don't panic. The weight will suddenly fall, and you'll be like one of the many people who ring me excitedly to say 'I'm eating like anything – and the weight's still dropping off!'

Once you have grasped the concept of my diet and exercise plan, you'll realize that you can eat absolutely anything you like, including chips, pastry and chocolate, as long as you stay within the portion control guidelines and never allow yourself to eat until bloated. *Never* treat a meal as if you won't get the chance to eat again. *Never* eat 'because it's been paid for'. Food is not your enemy, but once the control goes, we can end up stuffing everything in sight 'because the damage is done'. Your flatter stomach, and all the good feelings that go with knowing you look good, will last a lot longer than that massive pizza you gave in to. Just keep telling yourself it's worth it!

Many of you will be women who suffer a big stomach problem without being overweight. Few people realize just how bad it is to exist on a diet of processed calorie- or fat-reduced items, and the effect they can have on their stomachs. And why should they? Learn to live a little and eat what everyone else is eating. Keep drinking the water, however boring you may find it. Eat every three hours. With time, you'll be able to eat those 'controversial' foods when you know you can relax and not be on show, and watch your diet for a couple of days before you need to wear a particularly slinky skirt or pair of trousers.

Remember to look after your posture too. Not only is good posture essential for the appearance of your stomach, it is youthful. Never neglect your posture, and set aside a few minutes every day to stand in front of a mirror to check how you are standing and sitting.

And finally, exercise! Once you get into it, you'll wonder why you didn't do it before. You can lose weight without exercising, and indeed many bedridden people have successfully followed my plan, but a firm stomach needs good muscle tone. Exercise is good for your beauty, too, and you'll be proud of yourself for taking the trouble just to do that extra walk, or go for a brisk cycle ride.

Surprise everyone. Say goodbye to yo-yo dieting. Feel confident about your stomach and have them talking about the change in you. You'll never regret it.

Good luck for the future!